CONTENTS

Contents

PUBLIC HEALTH IMPACT OF PESTICIDES USED IN AGRICULTURE

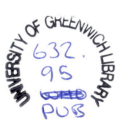

WORLD HEALTH ORGANIZATION
GENEVA
1990

WHO Library Cataloguing in Publication Data

Public health impact of pesticides used in agriculture.
  1. Pesticides – adverse effects   2. Pesticides – poisoning
  ISBN 92 4 156139 4   (NLM Classification: WA 240)

TYPESET IN INDIA
PRINTED IN ENGLAND

90/8430 — Macmillan/Clays — 4500

PREFACE

Concern about the effects of pesticides on health has been voiced in a number of reports, and activities to prevent such effects are carried out in most countries and at an international level. As pesticides are inherently toxic to living organisms, they are more likely to affect the health of human beings than other agricultural chemicals. However, the toxicity for human beings of different pesticides varies greatly and adverse affects on health may be prevented by choosing the least toxic pesticide, as well as by measures to reduce human exposure. The users of pesticides in agriculture have an obligation to prevent any adverse side-effects on health.

Even though a number of studies have been carried out on the problems of acute occupational, accidental, and suicidal poisonings by pesticides, there is a general lack of epidemiological data on the impact of pesticides on human health. Some follow-up studies of workers occupationally exposed to these chemicals have looked for chronic effects, but, because of methodological difficulties, the number of epidemiological studies of such effects has been small. Similarly, while exposure data are available for some populations (e.g., the occurrence of certain pesticides in human milk), there are few evaluations of the long-term effects.

The objective of the present publication is to assess the scope and severity, globally and regionally, of exposure to pesticides, to estimate future trends, and to review the effects of pesticides on human health, with particular reference to the general population in developing countries. The assessment is based primarily on published reports of the health effects of individual pesticides and on data collected by WHO and by UNEP (through the International Register of Potentially Toxic Chemicals). Most of the published reviews refer to the lack of information and the need for further epidemiological research on human exposures and health effects, and these shortcomings will naturally limit the scope of the present review.

This report is intended for use principally by the national health officials responsible for pesticide management and by research workers interested in the epidemiology of pesticide poisoning. Legislators, officers responsible for enforcing national regulations, and personnel involved in designing, developing, and implementing training programmes concerned with the health of agricultural workers and environmental protection will also find useful information in the report.

*

*   *

A preliminary draft of the report was prepared by: Dr U. Ahlborg, Toxicology Unit, National Institute of Environmental Medicine, Stockholm, Sweden; Dr M. Akerblom, National Laboratory for Agricultural Chemistry, Uppsala, Sweden; Dr G. Ekström, National Food Administration, Uppsala, Sweden; Dr C. Hogstedt, National Institute of Occupational Health, Solna, Sweden; Dr T. Kjellström, Division of Environmental Health, World Health Organization, Geneva, Switzerland; and Dr O. Pettersson, University of Agricultural Sciences, Uppsala, Sweden. This draft was then revised by a WHO/UNEP Working Group, which met in Tbilisi, USSR, on 23–27 November 1987. The members of the Working Group are listed below.

Funds for the preparation of the report and for the Working Group meeting were provided by the Swedish National Board of Occupational Safety and Health, UNEP, and WHO. The Institute of Sanitation and Hygiene of the Georgian Soviet Socialist Republic kindly hosted the meeting and all practical arrangements were made by the USSR Centre for International Projects. Valuable contributions to the text of the report were received from many staff in FAO, UNEP, and WHO, and from the International Group of National Associations of Manufacturers of Agrochemical Products.

WHO/UNEP Working Group on Public Health Impact of Pesticides Used in Agriculture

Dr U. Ahlborg, Toxicology Unit, National Institute of Environmental Medicine, Stockholm, Sweden

Dr M. Akerblom, National Laboratory for Agricultural Chemistry, Uppsala, Sweden

Dr W. Almeida, National Institute of Health Control, INCQS/FIOCRUZ, Rio de Janeiro, Brazil

Dr G. Ekström, National Food Administration, Uppsala, Sweden

Dr C. Hogstedt, National Institute of Occupational Health, Solna, Sweden (*Chairman*)

Dr M. Jaghabir, Department of Community Health, Jordan University, Amman, Jordan

Dr J. Jeyaratnam, Department of Community, Occupational and Family Medicine, National University of Singapore, Singapore

Dr F. Kaloyanova, Institute of Hygiene and Occupational Health, Sofia, Bulgaria

Dr T. Kjellström, Division of Environmental Health, World Health Organization, Geneva, Switzerland (*Secretary*)

Dr R. Levine, Nassau County Department of Health, New York State Department of Public Health, Mineola, NY, USA

Dr N. Maizlish, Occupational Health Surveillance and Evaluation Program, Berkeley, CA, USA

Dr G. Molina, Pan American Center for Human Ecology and Health, World Health Organization, Metepec, Mexico

Dr D. Mowbray, South Pacific Regional Environment Programme, Biology Department, University of Papua New Guinea, Waigani, Papua New Guinea

Dr J. N'Kurlu, Factories Inspectorate, Ministry of Labour and Manpower Development, Dar-es-Salaam, United Republic of Tanzania

Dr O. Pettersson, University of Agricultural Sciences, Uppsala, Sweden

Dr V. Polchenko, Laboratory of Systems Analysis of Public Health, Institute of Hygiene and Toxicology of Pesticides, Polymers, and Plastics, Kiev, USSR (*Vice-Chairman*)

Dr Y. Kagan, Chief, Department of Experimental Toxicology, Institute of Hygiene and Toxicology of Pesticides, Polymers, and Plastics, Kiev, USSR

Dr F. Xu, Institute of Environmental Health Monitoring, Beijing, China

Chapter 1

INTRODUCTION

What is a pesticide?

Most pesticides are chemicals that are used in agriculture for the control of pests, weeds, or plant diseases. These chemicals may be extracted from plants or may be "synthetic". This report will deal with those synthetic pesticides that represent potential hazards to public health.

FAO (1986a) defined a pesticide as any substance or mixture of substances intended for preventing, destroying, or controlling any pest, including vectors of human or animal disease, unwanted species of plants or animals causing harm during, or otherwise interfering with, the production, processing, storage, transport, or marketing of food, agricultural commodities,[1] wood and wood products, or animal feedstuffs, or which may be administered to animals for the control of insects, arachnids, or other pests in or on their bodies. The term includes substances intended for use as a plant-growth regulator, defoliant, desiccant, fruit-thinning agent, or an agent for preventing the premature fall of fruit, and substances applied to crops either before or after harvest to prevent deterioration during storage or transport. Similar definitions have been adopted by the Codex Alimentarius Commission (Codex, 1984) and the Council of Europe (1984). In each case, the term excludes fertilizers, plant and animal nutrients, food additives, and animal drugs.

Some pesticides are used both in agriculture and as vector control agents in public health programmes. Agriculture and horticulture, together with vector control programmes, account for the greatest use of pesticides. Significant amounts are also used in forestry and livestock production.

Some pesticides are of biological origin. One example is *Bacillus thuringiensis*, which is used in public health programmes to control mosquitos that transmit malaria and

---

[1] The term "agricultural commodities" refers to commodities such as raw cereals, sugar beet, and cottonseed, that might not normally be considered as food.

Simulium sp., the vector of onchocerciasis (river blindness), as well as in agriculture against lepidopteran pests.

Most pesticide preparations include carrier substances in addition to the active ingredients and also solvents and compounds that improve absorption, etc. These "inert ingredients" are not usually included in any discussion of the effects on health although they frequently comprise a large part of a commercial pesticide product, and their adverse effects may exceed those of the active ingredients. For example, carbon tetrachloride and chloroform, both potent agents that are toxic to the liver and central nervous system, may be used as "inert" ingredients without being mentioned on the product label. The adverse effects of pesticides on health may also be caused by impurities, such as dioxins in certain phenoxyacid herbicides, ethylene thiourea in ethylene bisdithiocarbamate fungicides, and isomalathion in malathion.

Types of exposure

Different groups and segments of a population are exposed to pesticides in different ways and in different degrees. Some exposures are intentional (suicides and homicides) and some are unintentional (Fig. 1).

Davies et al. (1980) and Davies (1984) described categories of pesticide exposure and the approximate size of the populations at risk in each case (Fig. 2). They used a triangle to represent the large population with low-level exposure, and a smaller group with extreme exposures. As will be discussed in Chapter 7, these relative population sizes do not necessarily reflect the number of poisonings that occur.

Fig. 1.   Types of exposure to pesticides

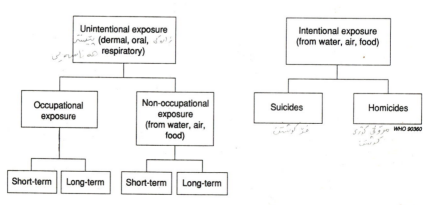

Fig. 2. Population groups at risk of exposure to pesticides[a]

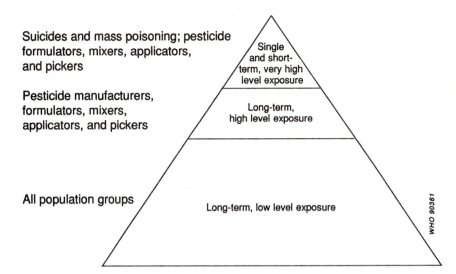

Suicides and mass poisoning; pesticide formulators, mixers, applicators, and pickers

Single and short-term, very high level exposure

Pesticide manufacturers, formulators, mixers, applicators, and pickers

Long-term, high level exposure

All population groups

Long-term, low level exposure

WHO 90361

The width of the triangle indicates the approximate size of the exposed groups

[a] Adapted from Davies et al. (1980) and Davies (1984).

Assessing the public health impact

Assessment of the public health impact of agricultural pesticides must include an estimation of the number of cases of severe and minor health effects, the number of fatalities and hospitalizations, and the effect on the health services of the treatments required. In some cases, sufficient data might be available to estimate the financial implications of the effects on the health services and the loss to society caused by the health effects. Any beneficial effects on health should be quantified in a similar way if possible.

A study of the indirect costs resulting from pesticide use in the United States of America (Pimentel et al., 1980) showed that they included: 45 000 nonfatal and fatal human cases of poisoning per year (the economic cost not estimated); US$ 12 million as a result of livestock losses; US$ 287 million as a result of a reduction in natural enemies and because of pesticide resistance; US$ 135 million resulting from honey-bee poisoning and reduced pollination; US$ 70 million as a result of losses of crops and trees; US$ 11 million as a result of fish and wildlife losses; and US$ 140 million from miscellaneous

13

losses. However, the 45 000 cases of poisoning and the US$ 839 million annual losses attributed to pesticide use may represent only a portion of the actual costs. Pimentel et al. (1980) pointed out that a more complete summation of the indirect costs would provide higher estimates. The purchase price of the pesticides used was estimated at US$ 2800 million and the estimated production benefits were US$ 10 900 million.

Thus the assessment of the public health impact is similar to environmental health impact assessment and to risk assessment. The items to be included are outlined in Table 1. In the following sections of this book, the available data on exposure to, and the health effects of, pesticides are analysed with these items in mind. Several of the items cannot be quantified because of lack of data.

Table 1. Factors to consider when estimating the impact of pesticide usage in agriculture on public health in developing countries

The total population at risk is divided into subpopulations with different average pesticide exposure levels:
— rural populations with traditional life-style and virtually no pesticide exposure;
— rural populations in areas with low use of pesticides;
— rural populations in areas with high use of pesticides, who are exposed through food, air, and water supply;
— rural populations in areas with high use of pesticides, additionally exposed via direct contact (for instance occupation);
— urban populations in areas with low use of pesticides on crops;
— urban populations in areas with high use of pesticides on crops;
— urban populations with additional direct contact exposure.

For each specific pesticide, the public health significance should be estimated, taking into account:
— effects on mortality in general;
— influence of mortality rates on productivity (need to take age-specific mortality into account);
— effects on overt disease morbidity (disease that disables the victim at least temporarily);
— influence of overt disease morbidity on occurrence of permanent disability;
— influence of overt disease morbidity on productivity (absence from work and daily duties);
— influence of overt disease morbidity on medical care services (staff use, drug use, bed use, costs);
— effects on the occurrence of lesser symptoms, and of physiological or biochemical changes;
— influence of these changes on sensitivity to other environmental factors, nutritional deficiencies, etc.

Chapter 2

PRODUCTION AND USE OF PESTICIDES

A short history

This short summary of the history of pesticide use is based on a review by Hassall (1982). The use of inorganic chemicals to control insects possibly dates back to classical Greece and Rome. Homer mentioned the fumigant value of burning sulfur, and Pliny the Elder advocated the insecticidal use of arsenic and referred to the use of soda and olive oil for the seed treatment of legumes. The Chinese were employing moderate amounts of arsenicals as insecticides by the sixteenth century and not long afterwards nicotine was used, in the form of tobacco extracts. By the nineteenth century, both pyrethrum and soap had been used for insect control, and also a combined wash of tobacco, sulfur, and lime to combat insects and fungi.

The middle of the nineteenth century marked the beginning of the first systematic scientific studies into the use of chemicals for crop protection. Work on arsenic compounds led to the introduction in 1867 of Paris green, an impure form of copper arsenite. It was used in the USA to check the spread of the Colorado beetle and by 1900 its use was so widespread that it led to the introduction of what was probably the first pesticide legislation in the world.

In 1896 a French grape grower, applying Bordeaux mixture (copper sulfate and calcium hydroxide) to his vines, observed that the leaves of yellow charlock growing nearby turned black. This chance observation demonstrated the possibility of chemical weed control, and shortly afterwards it was found that iron sulfate, when sprayed on to a mixture of cereal and weeds, killed the weeds without damaging the crop. Within a decade several other inorganic substances had been shown to act selectively at appropriate concentrations. Another important landmark was the introduction of the first organomercury seed dressings in 1913 in Germany.

In the years between the First and Second World Wars, both the number and the complexity of chemicals for crop protection increased. Tar oil was, and still is, used to control the eggs of aphids on dormant trees. Dinitro-orthocresol was patented in France in 1932 for the control of weeds in cereals, and in 1934 thiram, the first of several dithiocarbamate fungicides, was patented in the USA.

During the Second World War, the insecticidal potential of DDT was discovered in Switzerland and insecticidal organo-phosphorus compounds were developed in Germany. At about the same time, work was in progress in the United Kingdom that was to lead to the commercial production of herbicides of the phenoxyalkanoic acid group. In 1945, the first soil-acting carbamate herbicides were discovered by workers in the United Kingdom and the organochlorine insecticide chlordane was introduced in the USA and in Germany. Shortly afterwards, the insecticidal carbamates were developed in Switzerland.

In the period from 1950 to 1955, urea derivatives were developed as herbicides in the USA, the fungicides captan and glyodin appeared, and malathion was introduced. Between 1955 and 1960, other new products included herbicidal triazines and quaternary ammonium herbicides. Dichlobenil, trifluralin, and bromoxynil were described between 1960 and 1965 and the systemic fungicide benomyl in 1968. The leaf-acting herbicide glyphosate was introduced soon afterwards.

During the 1970s and 1980s many new pesticides were intro-duced. They have been based on a more thorough under-standing of biological/biochemical mechanisms, and they are often more effective at lower doses than the older pesticides. The best examples of this new generation of pesticides are the herbicidal sulfonylureas and the new systemic fungicides, such as metalaxyl and triadimefon. A new and important group of insecticides comprises synthetic light-stable pyrethroids, which have been developed from the naturally occurring pyrethrins.

As a result of a better knowledge of host–pest interactions, a new approach to the design of pesticides is now being devel-oped, as well as new strategies for formulations, and new methods of application. These developments provide an opportunity to reduce the risk of pesticide poisoning. The potential usefulness of microbial and other biological pest control agents is at present being studied by several research institutions around the world.

Classification of pesticides

Pesticides can be classified in many different ways: according to the target pest, the chemical structure of the compound used, or the degree or type of health hazard involved. Many authors, for example Hayes (1982) and Ware (1983), have developed systems of classification. A combined functional and chemical classification by Gunn & Stevens (1976) is given in Table 2.

Table 2. Classification of pesticides[a]

Main groups	Subgroups	Examples
Insecticides		
Inorganic		aluminium phosphide, calcium arsenate
Botanical (plant extracts)		nicotine, pyrethrin, rotenone
Organic	Hydrocarbon oils	citrus spray oils, dormant sprays ("winter washes"), mosquito larvicides
	Organochlorines	aldrin, BHC, DDT, heptachlor, toxaphene
	Organophosphorus compounds:	
	Non-systemic	azinphos methyl, dichlorvos, parathion, methyl parathion, fenitrothion, malathion
	Systemic	demeton methyl, dimethoate, monocrotophos, phosphamidon
	Carbamates	
	Non-systemic	carbaryl, methomyl, propoxur
	Systemic	aldicarb, carbofuran
	Synthetic pyrethroids	allethrin, bioresmethrin, permethrin
Microbial	Bacterial	*Bacillus thuringiensis*
	Viral	polyhedral viruses
Other insect-control agents		
Chemosterilants		apholate, metepa, tepa
Pheromones (sex attractants and synthetic lures)		
Repellents		deet, dimethyl phthalate, ethyl hexenediol
Insect hormones and hormone mimics (insect growth regulators)	Juvenoids (juvenile hormone mimics)	farnesol, methoprene
	Moulting inhibitors	diflubenzuron, ecdysone

17

Table 2   (continued)

Main groups	Subgroups	Examples
Specific acaricides		
Non-fungicidal	Organochlorines	chlorobenzilate, dicofol, tetradifon
	Organotins	cyhexatin
Fungicidal	Dinitro compounds	binapacryl, dinocap
	Other	chinomethionate
Protectant fungicides		
Inorganic		Bordeaux mixture, copper oxychloride, sulfur
Organic	Dithiocarbamates	mancozeb, metiram, propineb, thiram, zineb
	Phthalimides	captafol, captan, folpet
	Dinitro compounds	binapacryl
	Organomercurials	phenyl mercury (acetate and chloride)
	Organotin compounds	fentin (acetate and hydroxide)
	Others	chinomethionate, chloro-thalonil, dichlofluonid, dichlone, dicloran, dodine, dyrene, glyodin
Eradicant fungicides	(chemotherapeutants)	
	Antibiotics	blasticidin, cyclohexamide, kasugamycin, streptomycin
	Morpholines	dodemorph, tridemorph
	Formylamino compounds	chloraniformethan, triforine
	Others	ethirimol, carboxin dioxide, benomyl, tiabendazole, thiophanate-methyl
Soil fumigants and nematocides		
Soil sterilants	Halogenated hydrocarbons	chloropicrin, methyl bromide
	Methyl isothiocyanate generators	dazomet, metham
	Others	carbon disulfide, formaldehyde
Fumigant nematocides	Halogenated hydrocarbons	DD, dichloropropene, ethylene dibromide
Non-fumigant nematocides	Organophosphorus compounds	dichlofenthion, fensulfothion, fenamiphos
	Carbamates	aldicarb, carbofuran
Herbicides		
Inorganic		sodium arsenite, sodium chlorate
Organic	Phenolics	bromofenoxim, dinoseb acetate, DNOC, nitrofen, PCP
	Phenoxyacids (hormone weedkillers)	CMPP, MCPA, 2,4-D, 2,4,5-T

Table 2   (continued)

Main groups	Subgroups	Examples
Herbicides, organic (continued)	Carbamates	asulam, barban, bendiocarb, carbetamide, chlorpropham, phenmedipham, propham, tri-allate
	Substituted ureas	diuron, fluometuron, linuron, metobromuron, monolinuron
	Halogenated aliphatics	dalapon, TCA
	Triazines	ametryn, atrazine, methoprotryne, simazine, terbutryn
	Diazines	bromacil, lenacil, pyrazon
	Quaternary ammonium compounds:	
	bipyridyls	diquat, paraquat,
	pyrazolium	difenzoquat
	Benzoic acids	chlorfenprop methyl, dicamba, 2,3,6-TBA
	Arsenicals	cacodylic acid, DSMA, MSMA
	Dinitroanilines	nitralin, profluralin, trifluralin
	Benzonitriles	bromoxynil, chlorthiamid, dichlobenil, ioxynil
	Amides and anilides	benzoylprop-ethyl, diphenamid, propachlor, propanil
	Others	aminotriazole, flurecol, glyphosate, picloram

Dessicants, defoliants, and haulm killers[b]

	Quaternary ammonium compounds (bipyridyls)	diquat, paraquat
	Phenolics	cacodylic acid, dinoseb, DNOC, PCP

Plant growth regulators

Growth promoters (auxins and auxin type)		gibberellic acid
Growth inhibitors (stem shorteners)	Quaternary ammonium compounds	chlormequat
Sprout inhibitors and desuckering agents	Carbamates	chlorpropham, propham
Fruit setting, ripening, flowering agents and latex stimulants	Ethylene generators	ethephon
	Others	dimas, glyphosine, naphthaleneacetic acid
Fruit drop induction (abscission agents)		cycloheximide

Rodenticides

Fumigants (space fumigants also used for rodent control)		aluminium phosphide, calcium cyanide, chloropicrin, methyl bromide

Table 2 (continued)

Main groups	Subgroups	Examples
Anticoagulants	Hydroxy coumarins	coumatetralyl, difenacoum, warfarin
	Indandiones	chlorophacinone, phenyl-methyl pyrozolone, pindone
Others	Arsenicals	"arsenious oxide", sodium arsenite
	Thioureas	antu, promurit
	Botanical	red squill, strychnine
	Others	norbormide sodium, fluoroacetate, vitamin D (calciferol), zinc phosphide
Molluscicides		
Aquatic	Botanical	endod
	Chemical	copper sulfate, niclosamide, sodium pentachlorophenate, trifenmorph
Terrestrial	Carbamates	aminocarb, methiocarb, mexacarbate
	Other	metaldehyde

[a] Source: Gunn & Stevens (1976). Reproduced by kind permission of the publisher.
[b] Although compounds in this category are also herbicides, they are here being used on the crop itself, and in such applications are sometimes included in the general term "plant growth regulators".

Use of pesticides in agriculture

Crops are affected by different pests and by competition from weeds. Several insects and other arthropods, fungi, molluscs, and bacteria attack crops and result in quantitative and qualitative losses; the degree of damage varies greatly in different climatic and agricultural regions. With the introduction of new plant species and cultivars in plantation and cash-crop farming, increased problems can occur in the new monocultures. During the last three decades, chemical control of pests and weeds aimed at minimizing losses has been introduced throughout the world. A wide range of insecticides, fungicides, molluscicides, bactericides, and herbicides, including fumigants, have become important in agriculture, mainly in the developed countries, but also increasingly in the developing countries, where organochlorine insecticides are still used, but are being replaced gradually by organophosphorus, carbamate, and pyrethroid insecticides. Another important area for use of insecticides is for the control of ectoparasites, e.g., cattle dip.

The losses of crops caused by pests are great in developed as well as developing countries. In North America, Europe, and Japan, losses are estimated to be in the range 10–30%, but in the developing parts of the world, they are substantially higher (Edwards, 1986). Crop losses due to pests and plant diseases of the order of 40% are common in these areas, and losses of as much as 75% have been reported (Table 3). One of the major pests responsible for the greatest losses is the locust.

Even greater and often more significant losses occur after the crop is harvested, caused by pests that attack the stored products, particularly in the tropics (UNEP, 1981; FAO, 1985a). Many insect pests tunnel into grains or beans, where it is virtually impossible to kill them with pesticides. Rats and mice also cause significant losses of stored products.

Pests do not affect only the quantitative yields of the crops. Both pre-harvest and post-harvest infestations seriously affect food and feed quality. Measures taken to minimize crop losses are therefore also likely to improve product hygiene and other qualitative characteristics.

The data available in various countries or regions (Table 4) show a correlation between pesticide use and crop yield. When the agricultural practices are good (including adequate use of fertilizers), increased pesticide use leads to increased crop yields; but above a certain level of pesticide use other factors become limiting. Hence the correlation is not directly proportional. For example, the ratio between pesticide use per unit area of land in Japan and Africa is 85, whereas the ratio between the corresponding crop yields is only 4.5.

Table 3. Estimated percentage losses of potential crop yield[a]

Crop	South America	Africa	Asia
Wheat	31	42	30
Rice	28	36	57
Maize	44	75	42
Sugar cane	44	67	71
Potatoes	44	62	49
Vegetables and pulses	30	39	36
Coffee	47	56	43
Cocoa	48	52	38
Soya beans	32	42	40
Copra	34	30	50
Cotton	42	45	36

[a] Source: Edwards (1986). Reproduced by kind permission of the publisher.

Table 4. Pesticide use and yields of major crops in certain countries and areas[a]

Country or area	Pesticide use (kg/ha)	Rank	Crop yield (tonne/ha)	Rank
Japan	10.8	1	5.5	1
Europe	1.9	2	3.4	2
United States of America	1.5	3	2.6	3
Latin America	0.22	4	2.0	4
Oceania	0.20	5	1.6	5
Africa	0.13	6	1.2	6

[a] Source: Edwards (1986). Reproduced by kind permission of the publisher.

Use of pesticides in public health programmes

Many of the most important human diseases in the tropics are transmitted by vectors or intermediate hosts, such as insects or molluscs, that can be killed with insecticides or molluscicides (WHO, 1984e). A recent review (Edwards, 1986) identified five main vector-borne diseases for which pesticides are used: malaria, filariasis, onchocerciasis, schistosomiasis, and trypanosomiasis.

Other vector-borne diseases that can be controlled by use of insecticides include dengue fever, dengue haemorrhagic fever and Japanese encephalitis (all spread by mosquitos), Chagas disease (transmitted by reduviid bugs), leishmaniasis (transmitted by sandflies), and louse-borne typhus. To some degree, biological methods can also be used to control disease vectors (WHO, 1982b).

A WHO study (Smith & Graz, 1984) showed that the greatest demand for pesticides in urban vector control was for insecticides, the commonest formulations used being emulsifiable concentrates or ultra-low-volume (ULV) concentrates. In urban areas, organochlorine pesticides are now little used. They have been replaced by pyrethrins, pyrethroids, and organophosphorus insecticides, such as chlorpyrifos, dichlorvos, fenitrothion, fenthion, malathion, and temephos (WHO, 1988a). The overall pesticide requirements for urban public health programmes are substantial, the annual cost being estimated at over US$ 100 million (Smith & Graz, 1984). Nevertheless, this is a small amount compared with the cost of pesticides used in agriculture (see p. 27).

In 1980, about 50 000 tonnes of pesticides were used for public health programmes in developing countries. It was estimated that such programmes accounted for about 10% of total pesticide use, the remainder being used mainly in agriculture (Smith & Lossev, 1981).

Alternative methods of pest control

Many pesticides are potentially very hazardous not only to human health, but also to other organisms in the environment (Edwards, 1983a). Damage to an ecosystem may in itself lead to reduced agricultural production, decreased quality of the environment, and also economic losses outside agriculture. The balance between the benefits of pesticide use and the negative side-effects must therefore be evaluated in each agricultural setting and in each vector control programme.

Resistance is one of the major problems that has resulted from sustained intensive use of pesticides (WHO, 1986b). In some areas, the agricultural use of pesticides has caused resistance that severely affects the public health use of the same materials. When resistance to a pesticide begins to develop, the immediate effect is often that more of the pesticide is used. This may lead to eradication of the natural enemies of the pest and eventually to a resurgence of the pest itself, or to hitherto innocuous insects becoming major pests (FAO, 1979).

Chemical methods are not the only methods of pest control and not necessarily the best. A number of different approaches have been used, including application of particular agricultural procedures, and use of pest-resistant varieties of crops. There are also several biological methods that involve the release of sterile insects or of bacteria that kill the pest species, or the controlled release of insects or animals that consume the pests but not the crop. Storage conditions strongly influence post-harvest losses (FAO, 1985a) and food irradiation techniques can be used in certain circumstances for the protection of stored food (WHO/FAO, 1988).

The concept of integrated pest management (IPM) (originally called "integrated pest control", IPC) was developed as a means of improving the efficiency of pest control while at the same time keeping the cost and environmental damage of the pest control methods to a minimum (FAO, 1967). IPM is now the recommended approach for pest control and includes different control methods as appropriate, taking into account the local conditions of agriculture and pest occurrence (see pages 92–93 for further details). The same basic approach as

23

that used for pest control in agriculture has been developed by the United Nations Environment Programme and WHO for public health programmes and is known as integrated vector control (WHO, 1983).

A report is available on the application of IPM to cotton production in Nicaragua (Swezey et al., 1986). The problems that result from a combination of different harmful factors in Nicaragua are discussed and it is clear that, from the economic point of view, IPM has been successful in reducing the impact of pests on cotton production.

None of the available methods of pest control will totally eliminate vector-transmitted diseases or the losses that occur in crop yield or during post-harvest storage. Some studies (Repetto, 1985) have shown that the use of pest-resistant varieties of rice increases yield about as much as does moderate pesticide application, and that heavy pesticide application provides little additional improvement in yield when pest-resistant varieties are used.

Production and consumption of pesticides

Pesticides are used throughout the world, the intensity of use depending on a number of factors, such as the dominant crops, stage of development of the country, climatic conditions, and prevalence of pests. Wachter & Staring (1981) studied the pattern of development of pesticide use in agriculture and defined five stages, from very low use to very high (Table 5). The different stages are associated to some extent with the general economic development of the country. However, in any one country, the different stages of pesticide use may be found at the same time in different regions.

Now, a sixth stage could be included, in which the amount of active ingredient used is lower than 100 g/ha, as a result of the introduction of a new generation of pesticides, such as chlorsulfuron and metsulfuron methyl.

While figures on the global production of pesticides in terms of sales value are abundant, information on production in terms of weight or volume of active ingredient is extremely scarce. Green et al. (1977) published a diagram showing the steady growth in manufacture between 1945 and 1975 (Fig. 3). More recent data are not freely available.

Table 5. General development pattern of use of pesticides in agriculture[a]

Variable	Stage I (very low)	Stage II (low)	Stage III (moderate)	Stage IV (high)	Stage V (very high)
Level of use of pesticides in agriculture	Less than 100 g of active ingredient per ha	Over 100 but below 500 g of active ingredient per ha	Over 500 but below 1000 g of active ingredient per ha	Over 1 kg but below 5 kg of active ingredient per ha	Over 5 kg of active ingredient per ha; reduction through IPM
Product range	Few products (<50)	Mainly long established cheap products (organochlorines, DDT, HCH, malathion); range: 50–100	Wider product range, more modern insecticides, some herbicides; range 100–250	Full product range: herbicides and fungicides important; range 250–500	Full product range: over 500
Development of local pesticide industry	Imports formulated products	Mainly imported formulated products, a few products formulated locally	Local formulation accounts for 40–70% of domestic supply	Mainly local formulation; if country size permits, some local manufacture also	Hardly any imports of formulated products
Distribution structure	Mainly through extension service or cooperatives	Mainly through extension service; turnover small, a few private retailers have pesticides as a sideline	Private retailers are more involved	Turnover high enough for specialized retail shops to develop	Fully developed specialized retail outlets
Regulatory infrastructure	Non-existent or essentials only	Still underdeveloped	Underdeveloped or developed but not adequately enforced	Developed or sophisticated	Sophisticated
Area under control	Less than 5%	About 5–20%	About 50%	50–90%	Over 90%
General level of agricultural development	Mainly subsistence farming	Mainly subsistence farming but some cash crops relatively important	Late development: average yields	Developed: high yields	Sophisticated optimum inputs: high yields

[a] Source: Wachter & Staring (1981). Reproduced by kind permission of the publisher.

Fig. 3. World production of formulated pesticides, 1945–1985[a]

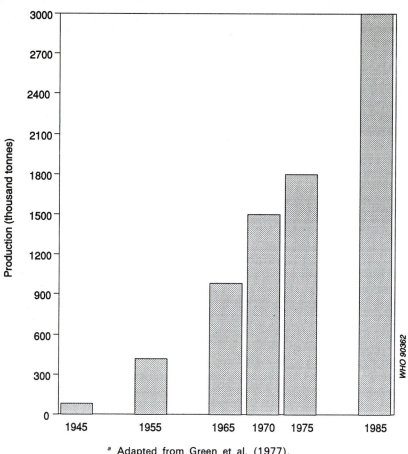

^a Adapted from Green et al. (1977).

The total sales of pesticides increased from US$ 3000 million in 1972 (Green et al., 1977) to US$ 15 900 million in 1985 (Table 6). The change in the value of the US dollar between 1972 and 1985 was 50.8:130.5 (base value 100 in 1980). Thus, the sum of US$ 3000 million in 1972 was equivalent to about US$ 7700 million in 1985. Thus, in real terms, the sales of pesticides doubled between 1972 and 1985. The actual increase is likely to have been somewhat less owing to increased sales of the more expensive new pesticides. Using this estimate, the global consumption of pesticides in 1985 would have been about 3 million tonnes (Fig. 3).

Another way of estimating the global use of pesticides is on the basis of the "market value" of agrochemicals as published, for instance, by Wood McKenzie & Co. (1987), or from the

Table 6. The value of the pesticide market in 1985 (million US$)[a]

Area	Herbicides	Insecticides	Fungicides	Others	Total
USA	3100	1090	330	330	4850
Western Europe	1475	850	1100	400	3825
East Asia	775	1300	785	90	2950
Latin America	485	655	250	60	1450
Eastern Europe	625	450	230	95	1400
Other	615	655	105	50	1425
World total	7075	5000	2800	1025	15900

[a] Source: Wood McKenzie Agrochemical Service (personal communication).

average price per tonne. Data are available only for exported pesticides (Wood McKenzie & Co. Ltd., personal communication), which had an average price in 1985 of US$ 5100/tonne. From the same report, the total market in 1985 can be estimated at US$ 15 900 million (Table 6). Thus, on the basis of export prices, the estimated number of tonnes used would be 3.1 million, very similar to the calculation above. According to data from Wood McKenzie & Co. Ltd., analysed by Mowbray (1988), 20% (equivalent to 600 000 tonnes annually) of the pesticides manufactured are exported to developing countries (Fig. 4).

The major groups of pesticides were used in 1985 in the following proportions: herbicides, 46%; insecticides, 31%; and fungicides, 18% (Anon, 1985). They were used on a number of different crops of different relative importance for world

Fig. 4. World pesticide market based on 1981 value (excluding non-crop outlets)[a]

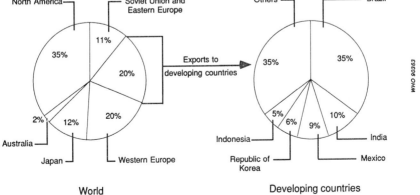

World

Developing countries

[a] From Mowbray (1988), based on Wood McKenzie Agrochemical Service data.

Table 7. Global production of major crops and the corresponding markets for herbicides, insecticides, and fungicides, 1985[a]

Crop	Production (million tonnes)	Pesticide market (million US$, 1984)		
		Herbicides	Insecticides	Fungicides
Sugar cane	941	148	42	26
Wheat	510	791	108	351
Corn, maize	490	1395	456	116
Rice	466	507	633	302
Potatoes	299	–	–	–
Sugar beet	283	287	97	49
Barley	178	–	–	–
Cassava (manioc)	137	–	–	–
Sweet potatoes	111	–	–	–
Soya beans	101	1348	128	28
Sorghum	77	102	56	12
Oats	46	–	–	–
Bananas	42	–	–	–
Coconuts	35	–	–	–
Millet	32	–	–	–
Rye	30	–	–	–
Groundnuts (peanuts)	21	46	65	55
Cotton	17	288	969	23
Fruits, vegetables, and horticultural crops	?	487	1168	1232

[a] Source: FAO (1986b), Anon (1985); cf. Tables A1.2, A1.3 and A1.4 in Annex 1.

agricultural production, as indicated in Table 7. It is seen that the greatest amounts of herbicides were used for corn and soybeans. The greatest amounts of insecticides were used on cotton and large amounts of fungicides were used on wheat and horticultural crops. A detailed analysis for different areas of the world (Anon, 1985) shows that about 75% of the total use was in Western Europe, Japan, and the United States of America.

Data on the consumption of individual pesticides in individual countries are extremely difficult to obtain, because manufacturers are reluctant to disclose such information. In addition, in many countries records are incomplete and there is little governmental control of the use of such chemicals. However, Annex 1 provides the data available for selected pesticides up to 1981.

According to Edwards (1986), overall pesticide use in agriculture, in terms of amounts applied per hectare, has been very much greater in Japan, Europe, and the United States of America than in the rest of the world, although China is also a major user. The fastest growing market, however, is Africa, with an increase in sales of 182% between 1980 and 1984. Other rapidly expanding markets are Central and South America (32% increase between 1980 and 1984), Asia (28%), and the Eastern Mediterranean region (26%). Although herbicide sales have been greater than those of insecticides and fungicides in developed countries and some developing countries and are increasing rapidly, this pattern is not being repeated in other developing countries, where insecticides still represent by far the greatest proportion of pesticides used. The pesticides most commonly used in certain Asian countries are listed in Table 8. This list includes some extremely hazardous pesticides (see Chapter 3).

It is difficult to interpret data from developing countries as different sources give different estimates. For instance, the total use of pesticides in Indonesia in 1978 is given as 4300 tonnes in one report (Balk & Koeman, 1984) and 13 400 tonnes in another (Staring, 1984). According to the latter report, the amount imported was 4300 tonnes. The use of pesticides can be presented on the basis of population or agricultural land area in order to facilitate comparisons. Such estimates (Table 9) show great differences among some Latin American countries.

Another factor of importance in assessing the potential public health impact of pesticides is the seasonality of their use. Each pest is of importance during only a limited part of the growing season and human exposure to pesticides is therefore also likely to be limited to the same periods. For example, in some parts of West Africa, herbicides and fungicides tend to be used early in the growing season, whereas insecticides are used at a later stage. This seasonality needs to be considered

Table 8. The fifteen most used pesticides in Bangladesh, India, Republic of Korea, Nepal, Pakistan, Philippines, and Thailand

1. carbaryl (I)	9. paraquat (H)
2. malathion (I)	10. aluminium phosphide (I)
3. parathion-methyl (I)	11. oxydemeton-methyl (I)
4. diazinon (I)	12. phosphamidon (I)
5. monocrotophos (I)	13. 2,4-D (H)
6. endosulfan (I)	14. BPMC (2-sec-butylphenyl methylcarbamate) (I).
7. carbofuran (I)	15. zinc phosphide (I)
8. mancozeb (F)	

I = insecticide   F = fungicide   H = herbicide.

Table 9. Use of pesticides in relation to population and agricultural land area (1982–84) in five Latin American countries[a]

Country	Population size (millions)	Agricultural area km²	Amount of pesticide used		
			tonnes	kg/person	kg/km²
Costa Rica	2.6	31 844	8 000	3.1	251
Guatemala	8.4	42 000	3 000	0.36	71
Colombia	29	310 000	21 000	0.72	68
Mexico	81	600 000	53 000	0.65	88
Brazil	136	1 200 000	42 000	0.31	35
World	4 000 000		2 000 000	0.5	

[a] Based on data published by Finkelman & Molina (1988).

in studies of acute human exposures and effects, as the figures for average annual exposure and incidence of poisoning may not reflect what is happening in the months of greatest pesticide use.

Future trends

The future use of pesticides will depend on several factors, including, of course, the need for pest control and the products available. Other factors are marketing, regulations, public attitudes, and the availability of alternative methods.

About 25% of the current world consumption of pesticides takes place in developing countries, mainly on cash-crops. As a country develops, the type and amounts of pesticides are likely to change from a small amount of organochlorine compounds used on a few crops to a wide range and larger total amounts of insecticides, fungicides, and herbicides on a large variety of crops. The present trend is for many crops to be treated with pesticides as soon as intensive land-use occurs. In some developing countries, the amounts of pesticide used currently far exceed the amounts used for the control of agricultural pests and diseases (Balk & Koeman, 1984).

As mentioned on p. 23, the incidence of pests and diseases in agriculture can be reduced by the proper management of naturally occurring regulatory mechanisms, but pesticides remain important additional tools even within this framework. The adoption of the principles of integrated pest management will lead to a reduced need for pesticides as compared with areas where pesticides are the only form of pest control employed.

Edwards (1986) published predictions of the future patterns of regional and national pesticide use, by class of pesticide and by type of crop. The following summary is based on his report. He suggested that future use would probably develop in line with expected changes in the relative importance of the crops, and that there might be a dramatic increase in pesticide use in developing countries, particularly in Africa (Table 10).

The organophosphorus compounds seem likely to continue to be the most important type of insecticide used in the developing countries and demand for them will probably more than double over the next ten years, but the more toxic of these chemicals will probably be phased out. Use of carbamates and pyrethroids is likely to increase substantially, while organochlorine use should decrease considerably. The amount of arsenical insecticides used will probably decline to a negligible level. There will be a considerable increase in the use of new products and non-chemical types of pest control.

Edwards predicted that the demand for both triazine and carbamate herbicides would probably treble by 1993, while that for phenylureas could more than double. There would probably be a substantial demand for chlorinated phenoxyacid compounds and for amides, if these were economically competitive. Although there could be some interest in newer types of weedkiller, the use of established products whose patents have expired is likely to show the greatest increase. It is unlikely that demand for herbicides will expand as rapidly in developing countries as in developed countries.

Edwards also predicted an increase in dithiocarbamate and phthalimide production. However, because these pesticides present several serious health problems, their use may actually

Table 10. Postulated percentage growth in pesticide use by region, between 1983 and 1993[a]

Region	1983–1988	1988–1993
Africa	60	200
Latin America	45	40
Eastern Mediterranean	25	22
East Asia	28	25
Other developing countries	15	12
All developing countries	37.5	55
World total	23	20

[a] Edwards (1986). Reproduced by kind permission of the publisher.

decrease. Mercury compounds are likely to be phased out completely in the next few years, while the organic, systemic fungicides will gain favour.

Any new types of chemical are likely to be less toxic and less persistent than existing ones. They will be developed for greater efficacy and selectivity, but are also likely to cost more. There are believed to be particularly good prospects for controlled-release compounds and naturally occurring (biological or chemical) pest control agents.

There should also be new developments in application techniques to suit local conditions in the developing countries. These will include improvements and modifications to conventional equipment to use smaller amounts of chemical, and greater use of integrated pest control systems.

As shown in Fig. 3, the use of pesticides approximately doubled every ten years between 1945 and 1975, and almost doubled again between 1975 and 1985 (see pages 24–26). Table 10 indicates that the use in developing countries is expected roughly to double again in the ten years from 1983 to 1993. If the public health problems associated with the use of pesticides are directly related to the amounts used, these figures may indicate the extent of future problems unless measures are taken to avoid or reduce the adverse health effects. About half of the increase in use of pesticides in developing countries will result from their application to a larger proportion of the agricultural land. The number of people exposed can be expected to increase accordingly. One indication of the association between pesticide use and public health problems is the WHO estimate of the number of cases of unintentional acute poisoning: half a million in 1972 and one million in 1985. This is the same rate of increase as that for estimated world consumption of pesticides.

Chapter 3

TOXIC EFFECTS OF PESTICIDES: EXPERIMENTAL AND CLINICAL DATA

The pesticides currently in use involve a wide variety of chemicals, as indicated in Table 2, with great differences in their mode of action, uptake by the body, metabolism, elimination from the body, and toxicity to humans.

With pesticides that have a high acute toxicity but are readily metabolized and/or eliminated, the main hazard is in connection with acute, short-term exposures. With others that have a lower acute toxicity but show a strong tendency to accumulate in the body, the main hazard is in connection with long-term exposure, even to comparatively small doses. Other pesticides that are rapidly eliminated but induce persistent biological effects, also present a hazard in connection with long-term, low-dose exposures. Adverse effects may be caused not only by the active ingredients and the associated impurities, but also by solvents, carriers, emulsifiers, and other constituents of the formulated product.

Acute toxic effects are fairly easily recognized, whereas the effects that result from long-term exposure to low doses are often difficult to distinguish. In particular, the effects of a regular intake of pesticide residues in food are hard to detect and quantify. Attempts to evaluate such effects are made regularly by the Joint WHO/FAO Meeting on Pesticide Residues (JMPR), which formulates recommendations on acceptable daily intakes (ADIs) and maximum residue limits (MRLs). The MRLs are usually used by the Codex Committee on Pesticide Residues (CCPR) in setting maximum residue limits (Codex MRLs) for pesticide residues on commodities in international trade.

It should be recognized that, for most pesticides, a dose–effect relationship has been defined, and that the effects of pesticides may be detected by measuring minor biochemical changes before adverse clinical health effects occur (Fig. 5). There may be a threshold below which no effects can be observed (no-observed-adverse-effect level). However, for pesticides that are

Fig. 5.   Manifestations of toxicant absorption[a]

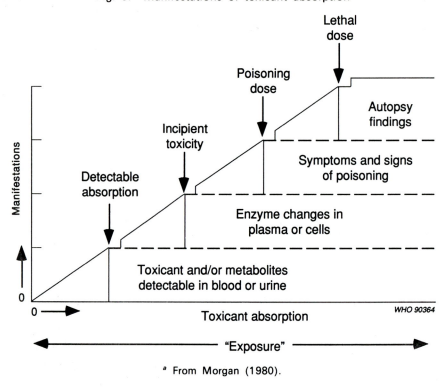

[a] From Morgan (1980).

suspected of causing cancer, the detection of early minor effects and the setting of no-observed-effect levels may not be relevant.

Factors influencing toxicity to humans

The severity of any adverse effects from exposure to a pesticide depends on the dose, the route of exposure, how easily the pesticide is absorbed, the types of effect of the pesticide and its metabolites, and its accumulation and persistence in the body.

The toxic effects also depend on the health status of the individual. Malnutrition and dehydration are likely to increase sensitivity to pesticides.

Pesticide uptake occurs mainly through the skin and eyes, by inhalation, or by ingestion. The fat-soluble pesticides and, to some extent, the water-soluble pesticides are absorbed through intact skin. Sores and abrasions may facilitate uptake through the skin (Table 11). Skin absorption is probably of particular

Table 11. Factors influencing skin absorption of pesticides

Skin characteristics	— sores and abrasions — wetness of skin — location on the body (absorption occurs readily through eyes and lips, for example) — vascularization
Environmental factors	— temperature — humidity
Pesticide characteristics	— acidity (pH) — vehicle — physical state (solid, liquid, gas) — concentration of active ingredient

importance when pesticides are used in developing countries, because adequate protective clothing is often not available or not worn (Jeyaratnam et al., 1987).

The vapours of pesticides or aerosol droplets smaller than 5 μm in diameter are absorbed effectively through the lungs. Larger inhaled particles or droplets may be swallowed after being cleared from the airways. Ingestion can also occur from the consumption of contaminated food or the use of contaminated eating utensils. Contaminated hands may also lead to intake of pesticides, for example from cigarettes.

Within the body, the pesticide may be metabolized, or it may be stored in the fat, or excreted unchanged. Metabolism will probably make the pesticide more water-soluble and thus more easily excreted. For instance, the fat-soluble pyrethroid insecticides are hydrolysed in the body to water-soluble substances, which are then excreted. Sometimes metabolism increases toxicity; for example, the hydrolysis of carbosulfan and furathiocarb produces the more toxic, and more water-soluble compound, carbofuran. Another example is the oxidation of the thiophosphorus insecticides to their oxygen analogues, which are much more potent inhibitors of the enzyme cholinesterase.

Some fat-soluble substances are not readily metabolized, but are stored in fatty tissues. Well known examples are the organochlorine compounds DDT and HCH. Such pesticides accumulate in the body and become more concentrated as they pass along the food chain. When they are stored in the fatty tissues, they are usually inactive. In times of poor nutrition or relative starvation, the deposits of fat are mobilized and the pesticides are released from these sites into the bloodstream, with the possibility of toxic effects if the concentration reaches a high enough level.

Interactions

The toxicity of pesticides may be influenced by environmental factors. In developing countries, where some people may suffer from nutritional deficiencies, for example protein deficiency, many pesticides have more severe toxic effects. The acute toxicity of pesticides is greater in rats fed on protein-deficient diets: for instance, the LD_{50} decreased 4-fold for DDT, 8-fold for carbaryl, 12-fold for lindane, 20-fold for endosulfan, and 2100-fold for captan (Almeida et al., 1978; Boyd et al., 1969, 1970; Krijnen & Boyd, 1970). Water deprivation may make people more susceptible to the effects of anticholinesterase pesticides (Baetjer, 1983). Hence, field workers suffering dehydration may be more susceptible to poisoning by organophosphorus and carbamate pesticides. A rise in ambient temperature, often makes the toxic effects of pesticides worse (Kagan, 1985).

When two or more pesticides are used simultaneously, they may interact and become either more toxic (synergism or potentiation, as with lindane and heptachlor) or less toxic (antagonism). Interactions of dietary nitrite with pesticides that contain a secondary amine group can result in the formation of nitrosamines, which may be more toxic, mutagenic, or carcinogenic. This effect has been demonstrated *in vitro* for 52 pesticides (Kearney, 1980). According to Kaloyanova (1983), interactions may occur after both short- and long-term exposure. Effects that result from the interaction of pesticides, although hard to quantify, are probably of more importance than is generally recognized.

Types of toxic effect

The mechanism of toxicity for mammals has been well characterized for only a few groups of compounds. For example, the mechanisms have been well defined for the organophosphorus and carbamate insecticides, both groups being inhibitors of cholinesterase, and for the nitrophenols and higher chlorinated phenols that are inhibitors of oxidative phosphorylation. The organomercury fungicides also have a well known mechanism of toxicity (WHO, 1976).

Some pesticides can be classified by their mechanism of toxicity (Kagan, 1985). Where this is not known, the pesticide may have to be classified by the symptoms it produces. Tables 12, 13, and 14 list important types of effect and relate them to particular groups of chemicals. In addition to the effects listed in these tables, high local exposures may cause "chemical burn" effects, the most serious being chemical burns to the eyes.

The International Agency for Research on Cancer (IARC) has evaluated the potential carcinogenicity of a number of pesticides; the information available is given in Table 15. IARC

Table 12. Recognized biochemical effects produced by certain pesticides

Effect	Mechanism and causative agent(s)
Enzyme induction	The induction of microsomal enzymes (mixed-function oxidases) in the liver is well known in experimental animals and in people treated with certain drugs or exposed to organochlorine pesticides. Occupational exposure increases the drug-metabolizing ability.
Enzyme inhibition	The inhibition of mixed-function oxidases of liver microsomes, e.g., aldehyde oxidase, by dithiocarbamates. Inhibition of blood cholinesterase by organophosphorus and carbamate insecticides is commonly detected, not only in cases of poisoning but also in workers exposed to the more toxic compounds of this group. Acute clinical poisoning is likely to appear when the cholinesterase activity is inhibited by 50% or more and 30% inhibition has been proposed as a "hazard level" (WHO, 1982a). Cumulative cholinesterase inhibition can occur following exposure to doses that do not produce clinical signs or symptoms; this depression lowers the threshold dose likely to produce clinical poisoning.

Table 13. Recognized skin effects of pesticides[a]

Effect	Causative agent(s)
Contact dermatitis	paraquat, captafol, 2,4-D, and mancozeb
Skin sensitization, allergic reaction, and rash	barban, benomyl, DDT, lindane, zineb, malathion
Photoallergic reactions	HCB, benomyl, zineb
Chloracne	organochlorine pesticides such as hexachlorobenzene, pentachlorophenol, and 2,4,5-T, probably as a result of contamination with chlorinated dioxins and/or dibenzofurans
Acquired toxic porphyria severe cutanea tarda manifestations, including photosensitivity, bulbae formation, deep scarring, permanent loss of hair, and skin atrophy)	hexachlorobenzene

[a] Source: W. F. Almeida (personal communication) and Bainova (1982).

Table 14. Recognized neurological effects of pesticides

Effect	Causative agent(s)
Delayed neurotoxicity	certain organophosphorus compounds, e.g., leptophos
Behaviour changes	certain organophosphorus insecticides
Lesions of the central nervous system	organochlorine and organophosphorus insecticides and organomercury fungicides
Peripheral neuritis	chlorophenoxy herbicides, pyrethroids and certain organophosphorus insecticides

has classified mineral oils (used as pesticides) as carcinogenic to human beings, and two pesticides—ethylene dibromide and ethylene oxide—as "probably carcinogenic to human beings". Fourteen pesticides were classified as "possibly carcinogenic to human beings": these were amitrole, Aramite, chlordecone, chlorophenols, chlorophenoxy herbicides, DDT, 1-3-dichloro-propene, hexachlorobenzene, hexachlorocyclohexanes, mirex, nitrofen, sodium orthophenylphenate, sulfallate, and toxaphene (IARC, 1988). None of the synthetic pesticides were classified by IARC as carcinogenic to human beings. The general lack of data from human studies is striking (Table 15).

A number of pesticides have been reported to be "carcinogenic to animals" (rats and mice) (Table 15) and these substances clearly represent a potential hazard to human beings.

Several short-term tests for mutagenicity have been proposed to detect potential chemical carcinogens. These short-term tests are useful for (a) predicting potential carcinogenicity in the absence of long-term tests of animal carcinogenicity, (b) deciding which chemicals should be tested or retested in animals, and (c) providing additional evidence to help with the interpretation of ambiguous data from experimental or epidemiological studies. Among the pesticides reviewed by IARC, ethylene dibromide and hydrazine (an impurity in maleic hydrazine) were considered as showing sufficient evidence of mutagenic acitivity in short-term tests to be classified as mutagenic. Kurinni & Pilinskaya (1976) estimated, on the basis of a literature review, that half of the 230 pesticides reviewed caused mutagenic effects.

Reproductive and other effects

An effect on human reproduction has been shown for dibromochloropropane (DBCP), which has produced sterility in males (see Chapter 4). Effects observed in animals include fetal

Table 15. IARC evaluations of evidence of carcinogenicity from animal and human studies of pesticides[a]

Pesticide[b]	Animal studies[c]				Human studies[d]			
	No evidence	Inadequate evidence	Limited evidence	Sufficient evidence	No evidence	Inadequate evidence	Limited evidence	Sufficient evidence
aldrin (5)			x			x		
amitrole (7, 41)				x		x		
Antu (30)		x			x			
Aramite (5)				x	x			
captan (30, S7)			x		x			
carbaryl (12)		x			x			
chlordane (20, 25, S7)			x		x			
chlordecone (20)				x	x			
chlordimeform (30, S7)		x				x		
chlorobenzilate (5, 30)			x		x			
p-chloro-o-toluidine (a metabolite of chlordimeform) (16, 30)				x	x			
chlorophenols (occupational exposure) (41)	x						x	
chlorophenoxy herbicides (occupational exposure) (41)	x						x	
chlorothalonil (30, S7)		x			x			
chlorpropham (12, S7)			x		x			
2,4-D and esters (15, S7)		x					x	
DDT (5, 7)				x		x		
diallate (12, 30)			x			x		
1,2-dibromo-3-chloropropane (15, 20, S7)				x	x			
1,2-dichloropropane (41)			x		x			
1,3-dichloropropene (41)				x	x			
dichlorvos (20, S7)		x				x		
dicofol (30)			x		x			
dieldrin (5)			x			x		
disulfiram (12, S7)		x			x			

Table 15 (continued)

Pesticide[b]	Animal studies[c]				Human studies[d]			
	No evidence	Inadequate evidence	Limited evidence	Sufficient evidence	No evidence	Inadequate evidence	Limited evidence	Sufficient evidence
endrin (5)		×			×			
ethylene dibromide (1,2-dibromo-ethane) (15)				×		×		
ethylene oxide (36, S7)				×			×	
ferbam (12, 13)		×			×			
fluometuron (30)		×			×			
heptachlor (5, 20, S7)			×		×			
heptachlor epoxide (5, 20)			×			×		
hexachlorobenzene (20, S7)			×[e]			×		
hexachlorocyclohexanes (5, 20, 32, S7)				×[f]		×		
malathion (30, S7)		×			×			
maneb (12)		×				×		
MCPA (30, S7)	×							
methoxychlor (5, 20, S7)		×					×	
methyl bromide (41)			×					
methyl parathion (30, S7)			(×)[g]		×			
mexacarbate (12, S7)		×[h]				×[h]		
mineral oils (S7)		×						×[i]
mirex (5, 20, 30)				×[i]	×			
monuron (12)			×					
nitrofen (30)				×	×			
parathion (30)		×			×			
pentachlorophenol (20, S7)		×					×	
phenoxyacid herbicides (occupational exposure) (S4)							×	
piperonyl butoxide (30, S7)		×			×			
propham (12)		×			×			
quintozene (5, S7)			×		×			
sodium ortho-phenylphenate (30, S7)				×	×			
sulfallate (30)				×	×			

2,4,5-T and esters (15, S7)
tetrachlorvinphos (30)

thiram (12, S7)
toxaphene (chlorinated camphenes) (20)
trichlorfon (30)
zineb (12, S7)
ziram (12, S7)

[a] Sources: IARC, 1974, 1976, 1977, 1979, 1982, 1983, 1985, 1987, and 1988.

[b] Reference to the appropriate volume number in the IARC Monographs series is given in brackets. S4 and S7 refer to IARC Monographs Supplement 4 (1982) and Supplement 7 (1988), respectively.

[c] The evidence of carcinogenicity in experimental animals was assessed and judged by IARC to fall into one of four groups, as follows:

(i) *Sufficient evidence* of carcinogenicity is provided when there is an increased incidence of malignant tumours: (*a*) in multiple species or strains; or (*b*) in multiple experiments (preferably with different routes of administration or using different dose levels); or (*c*) to an unusual degree with regard to incidence, site or type of tumour, or age at onset. Additional evidence may be provided by data on dose-response effects.

(ii) *Limited evidence* of carcinogenicity is available when the data suggest a carcinogenic effect but are limited because: (*a*) the studies involve a single species, strain or experiment; or (*b*) the experiments are restricted by inadequate dosage levels, inadequate duration of exposure to the agent, inadequate period of follow-up, poor survival, too few animals, or inadequate reporting; or (*c*) the neoplasms produced often occur spontaneously and, in the past, have been difficult to classify as malignant by histological criteria alone (e.g., lung adenomas and adenocarcinomas, and liver tumours in certain strains of mice).

(iii) *Inadequate evidence* of carcinogenicity is available when, because of major qualitative or quantitative limitations, the studies cannot be interpreted as showing either the presence or absence of a carcinogenic effect.

(iv) *No evidence* of carcinogenicity applies when several adequate studies have shown that, within the limits of the tests used, the chemical or complex mixture is not carcinogenic.

[d] The evidence for carcinogenicity from studies in human beings was assessed and judged by IARC to fall into one of four groups, defined as follows:

(i) *Sufficient evidence* of carcinogenicity, i.e., there is a causal relationship between exposure and human cancer.

(ii) *Limited evidence* of carcinogenicity, i.e., a causal interpretation is credible, but that alternative explanations, such as chance, bias or confounding, cannot be excluded.

(iii) *Inadequate evidence* of carcinogenicity, which applies to both positive and negative evidence, indicates that one of two conditions prevailed: (*a*) there are few pertinent data; or (*b*) the available studies, while showing evidence of association, do not exclude chance, bias or confounding.

(iv) *No evidence* of carcinogenicity applies when several adequate studies have shown no evidence of carcinogenicity. It should be noted that the categories "sufficient evidence" and "limited evidence" refer only to the strength of the experimental evidence that these chemicals or complex mixtures are carcinogenic and not to the extent of their carcinogenic activity nor to the mechanism involved. The classification of any chemical may change as new information becomes available.

[e] β and γ isomers.　　[f] Technical grade and α isomer.　　[g] Evidence suggesting lack of carcinogenicity in animal studies.　　[h] Highly refined oils.　　[i] Untreated and mildly treated oils.

41

death and absorption attributable to 2,4,5-T contaminated by 2,3,7,8-tetrachlorodibenzo-*p*-dioxin. Teratogenicity or fetal toxicity has been reported in at least some mammalian species for the following pesticides: carbaryl, captan, folpet, difolatan, organomercury compounds, 2,4,5-T, pentachloronitrobenzene, paraquat, maneb, ziram, zineb, and benomyl.

Effects on the reproductive system of female animals have been reported for chlordecone, thiram, and ziram (Kagan, 1985).

Pesticide-induced teratogenicity and its relationship to human health must be considered from a dose–effect standpoint. In experimental studies, the effects were usually dose-dependent and the doses required to produce teratogenic effects were generally far in excess of those that human beings might be expected to receive under normal conditions.

Other recognized effects of pesticides include:

— cataract formation, caused by exposure to diquat;
— cellular proliferation in the lungs, caused by paraquat (WHO, 1984c);
— effects on the immune system, caused by dicofol, organotin compounds, and trichlorfon;
— uncoupling of oxidative phosphorylation, caused by dinitrophenols and dinitrocresols, for example (Weinbach, 1957).

Quantitative aspects of toxicity and risk classification

Ideally, the human dose–effect and dose–response relationships should be known for each pesticide in order to be able to establish safety standards and to classify them according to the degree of health risk. For most pesticides, these relationships are not known and preventive measures have therefore been developed on the basis of the LD_{50} and other crude measures of the dose–response relationship in animals.

WHO (1990) and the Council of Europe (1984) have grouped formulated pesticides by degree of hazard (Table 16) and the "hazard class" of a pesticide has now been incorporated into legislation in many countries. Some countries, e.g., Bulgaria (Kaloyanova, 1982, 1986) and the USSR (Kagan, 1985) have developed their own classification (Table 17).

Table 16. Classification of pesticides according to degree of hazard to human beings

| Hazard class | | LD$_{50}$ (rat) (mg/kg of body weight)[a] | | | |
| | | Oral | | Dermal | |
		Solid[b]	Liquid[b]	Solid[b]	Liquid[b]
Ia	Extremely hazardous	5 or less	20 or less	10 or less	40 or less
Ib	Highly hazardous	5–50	20–200	10–100	40–400
II	Moderately hazardous	50–500	200–2000	100–1000	400–4000
III	Slightly hazardous	over 500	over 2000	over 1000	over 4000

[a] A dosage of 5 mg/kg of body weight is equal to a few drops ingested or a splash in the eye, 5–50 mg/kg of body weight equals up to one teaspoonful, and 50–500 mg/kg of body weight corresponds to up to two tablespoonfuls.
[b] The terms "solid" and "liquid" refer to the physical state of the product or formulation being classified.

Copplestone (1982) reviewed the distribution of technical pesticides among the various hazard classes. Many of the organophosphorus insecticides were considered to be very hazardous. The uses and choice of selected individual pesticides, based on recommended restrictions on availability, are shown in Annex 2.

Certain countries have moved some pesticides between categories on the basis of problems peculiar to them; for example, in Malaysia paraquat has been moved from hazard class II to Ib.

Table 17. Classification of pesticides by toxicity in Bulgaria[a]

Factor	Extremely hazardous	Highly hazardous	Moderately hazardous	Slightly hazardous
Oral LD_{50} for rat: liquid solid	<50 mg/kg <10 mg/kg	50–100 mg/kg 10–30 mg/kg	100–1000 mg/kg 30–300 mg/kg	>1000 mg/kg >300 mg/kg
Percutaneous LD_{50} for rat: liquid solid	<100 mg/kg <30 mg/kg	100–500 mg/kg 30–150 mg/kg	500–2000 mg/kg 150–600 mg/kg	>2000 mg/kg >600 mg/kg
LC_{50} for rat, (inhalatory, 4 hr exposure)	<200 mg/m³; saturation concentration is above toxic level; provokes severe acute poisoning	200–1000 mg/m³; saturation concentration is above threshold level; provokes poisoning	1000–5000 mg/m³; saturation concentration causes slight effect and is about equal to threshold level	>5000 mg/m³; saturation concentration provokes no effect
Coefficient of cumulation (K)[b]	K<1	1≤K<3	3≤K≤5	K>5
Persistence in environment: period of decomposition (half-life)	Quite persistent: above 1 year	Persistent: 6–12 months	Moderately persistent 1–6 months	Slightly persistent under 1 month
Carcinogenicity	Proved human carcinogen; strong carcinogen for test animals	Slightly carcinogenic for test animals; cancer in <20% of the animals with maximum non-toxic doses; suspected human carcinogen	No carcinogenic effect	No carcinogenic effect
Teratogenicity	Proven human abnormalities, reproducible in test animals; teratogenic activity with doses met in practice	Strong teratogen; 50–100% response in test animals at doses not toxic for mother; effect with more than one type of test animal; polytropic adverse effect	Abnormalities in fewer than 50% of offspring at doses not toxic for mother; teratogenic effect in one type of test animal; affects single organs and systems; effective dose above 1/10 LD_{50}	No teratogenicity
Embryotoxicity	Not recorded in assessment	Selective embryotoxicity at doses not toxic for mother	Moderate embryotoxicity at doses toxic for mother	No embryotoxicity effect

	Acute severe poisonings possible in practical application	Probable acute poisonings	Acute poisonings only in exceptional conditions	Acute poisonings not probable
Severity of human poisoning				
Therapeutic possibility	No special treatment; poor therapeutic possibility	Antidotes available; fair therapeutic possibility	Antidotes available; good therapeutic possibility	Specific treatment: good therapeutic possibility
Irritation of skin	Very strong irritant; chemical burning; acute toxic dermatitis from concentrated preparations; toxic dermatitis from field formulations	Strong irritant; rapid development of symptoms; toxic dermatitis from concentrated preparations; cumulative effect of field formulations	Irritant; cumulative dermatitis from concentrated preparations	Practically nonirritating
Irritation of eyes and upper respiratory organs	Field formulations have irritant effect	Field formulations have slightly irritant effect	Concentrated preparations have irritant effect	No practical irritant effect of even concentrated preparations
Allergies; sensitization	Established allergic and photosensitizing effect in humans; positive evidence of sensitization of guinea pigs.	Established allergic effect in humans; negative sensitizing test in guinea pigs	Presumed sensitizing effect on basis of chemical structure	No sensitizing effect

Notes

1. When decisions on preliminary control are being made, some pesticides may be put in an adjacent class of hazard. In addition to the limiting criteria, the remaining toxicological properties, type of sensitivity, type of formulation, and economic importance are considered in the first assessment.

2. If the practical application of pesticides indicates that conditions for creating vapours, liquids or solid aerosols of the preparation are possible, the criterion for inhalation toxicity is taken as limiting.

[a] Source: Kaloyanova (1986). Reproduced by kind permission of the publisher.

[b] $K = \dfrac{LD_{50} \text{ (chronic exposure)}}{LD_{50} \text{ (acute exposure)}}$

Chapter 4

SHORT- AND LONG-TERM HEALTH EFFECTS OF PESTICIDES: EPIDEMIOLOGICAL DATA

Very limited epidemiological data are available for evaluation of the health effects of pesticides on humans; this is surprising and gives rise to concern in view of the very high toxicity and potential health risk of certain products. The most complete collection of published reports is that prepared by Hayes (1982). Some cases of severe mass poisoning are described below, but these are rare occurrences in relation to the widespread use of pesticides. Scattered individual cases of poisoning have been discovered from hospital records in some countries, but few reports are available that analyse the overall situation in countries or districts. This may be because the effects are not recognized by health workers as being due to pesticides, because they are not reported or published even if recognized, or because the effects truly do not occur. Only intensified efforts to monitor the use of pesticides, human exposures, and health effects will be able to identify the reason.

It should be emphasized that the results of surveys of the health effects of pesticides that do not show any clear effects are often not published, because scientists and journals are reluctant to report "negative" findings. Thus, there may be more data available showing the absence of effects than the published reports indicate. These "negative" reports are, in fact, just as important as the positive ones.

Only a small proportion of a population is likely to receive a pesticide dose high enough to cause acute severe effects; but many more may be at risk of developing chronic effects, depending on the type of pesticide they are exposed to. In order to demonstrate the occurrence of the different types of effects in a population, the first step should be to study the distribution of the different levels of exposure.

Epidemiological studies of low-dose groups are difficult because the chronic effects are often not specifically associated with pesticide exposure and the exposure or dose levels are often difficult to measure. In addition, since the effects being sought, for instance cancer or chronic neurological disease, are usually rare, any cohort epidemiological study in low-dose groups needs to be very large in order to produce meaningful results. Smaller-scale case–control investigations, however, have proved to be a valid alternative (Zielhuis, 1972).

The individuals who receive very high doses usually belong to well defined groups, for example people using pesticides under primitive field conditions with insufficient protective equipment and training, people attempting to commit suicide with pesticides, or people accidentally exposed through consuming highly contaminated food or beverages. Epidemiological studies of such groups are available and give detailed descriptions of the acute health effects observed. In many cases, however, the quantification of the exposure and dose is given in less detail as the studies are often initiated only after the effects have been observed. At the time the study starts, the data on previous exposures may be difficult to collect. Nevertheless, epidemiological studies of people who have been exposed to high doses (usually through occupational exposure) are of great value in indicating the "upper limit" of effects that could possibly occur (Zielhuis, 1972). In addition, effects that take a long time to develop in low-dose groups may occur more rapidly in the high-dose group and these effects may be preceded by early subclinical effects that can be studied over a period of time.

In the following sections the effects of pesticides will be discussed in relation to the different types of intentional and unintentional exposure (see Fig. 1, p. 12). In order to get an overview of the reported human health effects, a summary table has been prepared for a number of the more widely used pesticides, using data from the WHO Environmental Health Criteria publications (Table 18). The lack of data is evident, and in those cases where suicide attempts or occupational or accidental exposure has led to human health effects, the exposures have usually been very high.

Intentional exposure

In several studies, it has been concluded that intentional poisonings (mainly attempted or successful suicides) make up a large proportion of the poisonings by pesticides of high toxicity, in certain developing countries. In Indonesia, Malaysia, and Thailand, for example, the proportion of acute

Table 18. Reported health effects in humans from selected pesticides after different types of exposure

Pesticide	Maximum acceptable daily intake (mg/kg of body weight)[a]	IARC evaluation number[a]	WHO/FAO data sheet number[a]	Environmental Health Criteria number[a]	Data on human effects reported in WHO Environmental Health Criteria[b]			
					Suicides	Occupation	Accidents	General environment or food
Aldicarb	0.005	N.A.	53	N.A.	0	(1)	(2)	0
Aldrin	0.0001	5	41	91	0	–	+	0
Campheclor	N.A.	20	20	45	+	–	+	0
Chlordane	0.0005	20	36	34	±		0	–
DDT	0.02	5, 7	21	9	0	(3)	(4)	0
Dieldrin	0.0001	5	17	91		(1)		
Endrin	0.0002	5	1	N.A.				
Ethylene dibromide	N.A.	15	N.A	N.A.				
Heptachlor	0.0005	5, 20	19	38	0	–	0	(5)
Lindane	0.01	5, 20	12	N.A.				
Mirex	N.A.	5, 20	N.A.	44	0	0	0	0
Paraquat	0.004	N.A.	4	39	+	±	+	0
Parathion	0.005	30	6	63	+	+	+	0
Pentachlorophenol	N.A.	20, 41	N.A.	71	+	+	+	±
2,4,5-T	0.03	15, 41	13	29	0	+ (6, 7)	0	0

[a] N.A. = not applicable.

[b] (1), no fatal cases; (2), no mass poisoning; (3), no effects, except dermatitis at high exposure; (4), 400 deaths due to contaminated water; (5), high levels in breast milk; (6), chloracne; (7), association with human cancer; 0, no data reported; +, data showing effects; –, data showing lack of effects.

pesticide poisonings that are suicide attempts has been reported to be 62.6%, 67.9%, and 61.4%, respectively (Jeyaratnam et al., 1987). When such compounds are easily available in many households, they may become the "method of choice" for individuals with suicidal intent. One of the few detailed studies of this problem was carried out in Sri Lanka (Jeyaratnam et al., 1982). Hospital records for 1975–80 were reviewed and it was found that in a total population of about 15 million people, there were on average 13 000 hospital admissions for pesticide poisoning each year, three-quarters as a result of suicide attempts. About 1000 of these patients died. The most common types of pesticide involved in the poisonings were organophosphorus compounds. The report concluded that the incidence of pesticide poisoning in 1979 was 79 per 100 000 population. The equivalent figure for suicide attempts using pesticides was 58 per 100 000 population. The other main causes of unintentional poisoning were occupational exposure (13 per 100 000) and accidental exposure (6 per 100 000).

Other detailed studies in Pacific island countries (Mowbray, 1986; Taylor et al., 1985) and elsewhere (WHO, 1984c) have documented the use of paraquat in many suicide attempts. In the WHO review 400 specific cases are referred to. The ingestion of a sufficient amount of paraquat will lead to irreversible fatal lung damage. An increased ratio of suicidal to accidental poisoning with this pesticide has been reported in some studies (WHO, 1984c). It is important to recognize that suicide attempts often represent a cry for help, and that the easy accessibility of highly toxic agents may mean that what was intended only as a gesture becomes a fatal event.

Cultural factors will influence whether suicide attempts and suicides are reported, and which method is used for a suicide attempt. The Sri Lankan experience may not be typical, but a study in Zimbabwe also reported a large proportion of suicide attempts among pesticide poisonings (Hayes et al., 1978).

No systematic population-based data on the role of pesticides in homicides are available but it is likely that highly toxic pesticides would be used by people with homicidal intent in countries where they are easily available.

Occupational exposure

Acute effects

A large number of reports are available on the acute effects associated with high occupational exposure to pesticides. These include reports of acute chemical burns of the eye, skin damage, neurological effects, and liver effects (see Chapter 3). A review of data on unintentional pesticide poisoning in 35 countries was prepared by Levine (1986). Some of the data originated from specific *ad hoc* studies, and some were taken from official national statistics of poisonings. The majority of cases of unintentional pesticide poisonings were of occupational origin, occurring largely among plantation workers and farmers mixing or using pesticides. In the Sri Lankan study referred to earlier (Jeyaratnam et al., 1982), about 70% of the unintentional poisonings were due to occupational exposure. Levine (1986) reported annual incidence rates of unintentional pesticide poisoning of between 0.3 and 18 per 100 000 from population-based studies in 17 countries. Longitudinal data on the incidence of poisoning in Thailand showed an increase from about 1 case per 100 000 population per year in the early 1970s to about 5 cases per 100 000 per year in the early 1980s. These studies are likely to refer mainly to acute cases of poisoning, as these would produce sufficiently severe and specific effects for the case to be recognized as pesticide poisoning. However, it has been proposed by Loevinsohn (1987) that deaths due to pesticide poisoning may be misclassified as "strokes" in communities with poor diagnostic facilities. Additional data (Polchenko, 1974), based on a survey of more than 50 000 cases throughout the world between 1945 and 1972, showed that most such poisonings were associated with highly toxic pesticides with LD_{50} of up to 50 mg/kg of body weight and a half-life in human tissues of more than one month.

The accuracy of the available data on pesticide poisonings depends on the ability of the investigators to document the exposures. Organochlorine pesticides accumulate in the body fat and can be measured a long time after exposure ceases (WHO, 1979, 1984b, 1984d), while organophosphorus pesticides (WHO, 1986c) and carbamates (WHO, 1986d, 1988b) reduce the activity of cholinesterase in red blood cells, which can be used as an indicator of current exposure. Many of the reports on acute poisoning deal with organophosphorus poisoning.

When an outbreak of mass poisoning occurs in a specific occupational group, the cases brought to the medical services with acute or fatal poisoning may lead to a systematic survey being carried out. One of the largest such surveys was among 7500 field workers engaged in malaria control in Pakistan (Baker et al., 1978). These workers were spraying a malathion formulation that had become partially converted to iso-malathion as a result of problems in production and storage. Poisonings started occurring soon after the beginning of the spraying programme, and five workers died. On the basis of questionnaires regarding symptoms, it was estimated that at least 2800 workers had been poisoned. Biochemical signs of poisoning were correlated with both the reports of symptoms and duration of exposure. Workers spraying DDT had no symptoms of poisoning. Baker et al. did not report the proportion of workers admitted to hospital, but it is likely that the vast majority of cases were only identified because of the systematic study. The case-fatality rate was about 0.2%, which can be compared with the rate of about 9% of hospital admissions in Sri Lanka (Jeyaratnam et al., 1982). On the basis of these reports, it can be estimated that for every 500 symptomatic cases, there are 11 hospital admissions and one death.

The extreme effects (death and hospitalization) are likely to be easier to study than symptoms, which require careful assess-ment using proper epidemiological methods. Biochemical effects require the systematic application of specific tests which are often not routinely available in the field. Even more difficult is testing for genetic effects, for example chromosomal aber-rations, which have been reported among pesticide workers with symptoms of poisoning (Dulout et al., 1985). In areas where organophosphorus pesticides are used extensively, the availability of facilities for cholinesterase testing is of great importance. Surveys with this test have helped identify popula-tions with significant exposure. The study in Pakistan (Baker et al., 1978) is one example. Another is a study of four Asian countries (Jeyaratnam et al., 1986), which showed that about 24% of 821 pesticide "users" in Malaysia and about 30% of 144 "users" in Sri Lanka had cholinesterase inhibition exceeding 25–30%. WHO (1982a) has proposed a "hazard level" of 30% inhibition (Table 12); in Thailand and Indonesia, fewer than 1% of the "users" had such reductions.

In a study of self-reported cases of pesticide poisoning and hospital admissions for poisoning (Jeyaratnam et al., 1987), about 7% of the agricultural workers in Malaysia and Sri Lanka who used pesticides were found to have been poisoned in the previous year. The proportion of occupational poisonings among the hospital admissions was 14–32%, non-occupational accidents about the same proportion, and most of the rest were suicides. Data on pesticide poisoning and cholinesterase inhibition among agricultural workers in Latin America (Finkelman & Molina, 1988) indicate that 10–30% of such workers in particular groups may be affected. In the USA, two separate surveys of pesticide poisonings among farm workers (Griffith et al., 1985; CDFA, 1986) each reported prevalences of confirmed cases of 2.2–16%.

A recent bibliography and review of the available reports on the health effects associated with environmental hazards in developing countries (WHO, 1987a) found that very few epidemiological studies had been properly performed. Most of the reports were reviews or commentaries or dealt only with either clinical evaluations or exposures. Such reports are available from several developing countries (Senewiratne & Thambipillai, 1974; Mackintosh et al., 1978; Kashyap, 1979; Wohlfart, 1981; Gupta et al., 1984; Singh & West, 1985; Baloch, 1985; Berger, 1988). Some studies of occupational exposures (e.g., Copplestone et al., 1976; Howard et al., 1981) showed that workers spraying pesticides who employ appropriate protective methods can prevent excessive exposures and the associated health effects. Other studies (e.g., Shih et al., 1985) have shown a reduction over time of the incidence of poisoning when preventive methods are introduced.

In the bibliography prepared by WHO (1987a), there were reports of occupational poisoning from all WHO regions and all continents. In view of the rapidly increasing use of pesticides in developing countries, it is clear that there is a great need for further studies in order to assess properly their public health impact.

Acute occupational exposure may also occur during the manufacture, formulation, packaging, and transport of pesticides, and among people re-entering a previously treated area.

Chronic effects

Bone marrow effects

Since 1948, there have been at least 30 reports involving 64 instances of aplastic anaemia and related blood dyscrasias associated with pesticides, many of which have occurred in people exposed in occupational settings. To date, however, the most likely explanation of these reports appears to be one of a rare idiosyncratic bone-marrow reaction to a pesticide in particular individuals (Hayes, 1982).

Cancer

The International Agency for Research on Cancer (IARC) has evaluated phenoxyacid herbicides, chlorophenols, 2,4-D, and 2,4,5-T and concluded that there is "limited evidence" of carcinogenicity for human beings (Table 15) as exposure to these compounds was found to be associated with soft-tissue sarcomas (IARC, 1988).

There is strong evidence that arsenical pesticides are associated with respiratory cancer in human subjects. Studies among pesticide packers in Baltimore, Maryland (USA), and Koblenz (Federal Republic of Germany) have demonstrated the importance of this factor among occupational groups. Nordberg & Andersen (1981), however, suggested that environmental exposure to arsenic is always coupled with exposure to other metals, sulfur dioxide, or organic carcinogens.

Evidence of carcinogenicity of organochlorine pesticides for human beings is not strong (Table 15). However, the persistence of these agents in the environment, the continued use of DDT in developing countries, and animal evidence consistent with carcinogenicity make further study imperative.

Several investigations of cancer among farmers and pesticide workers have indicated increased risk. While impressed with the general consistency of these studies, Sharp et al. (1986) were nevertheless cautious in interpreting them. Specifically, they argued that while the outcome in these investigations was generally derived on an individual basis, the measures of exposure came either from indirect data (e.g., occupation) or from group summary data (e.g., usage).

Reproductive effects

Male infertility has been observed in association with exposure to the nematocide dibromochloropropane (DBCP) (Wharton et al., 1977, 1979). As regards reproductive effects related to the phenoxy herbicides and their contaminants, there have been many investigations, but little consistency in the results. This inconsistency may reflect the fact that the effects observed at exposure levels commonly experienced by human beings are weak. Other methodological difficulties (e.g., with follow-up) may also have contributed to the problems associated with these studies.

Cytogenetic effects

Although data are scarce, almost all reports of cytogenetic damage associated with pesticide exposure have come from occupational studies. The earliest report by Yoder et al. (1973) found increased chromosomal damage among herbicide and insecticide sprayers during the peak spraying season. However, the frequency of damage was lower among sprayers than among controls in the off season; it has been pointed out (Friedman, 1984) that the histological slides of the chromosomes were not read blindly in this study. Nevertheless, there have been confirmatory reports by Rabello et al. (1975) regarding workers producing DDT, and by Dulout et al. (1985) with reference to flower growers exposed to organophosphorus compounds, carbamates, and organochlorines. In contrast, Steenland et al. (1985) did not find cytogenetic effects among forestry workers exposed to phenoxyacid herbicides and sprayers using ethylene dibromide.

Neurotoxicity

The chlorinated hydrocarbon insecticide chlordecone was responsible for more than 57 cases of neurological disease among workers in Hopewell, Virginia, in 1975 (Taylor et al., 1976). Several workers continued to manifest signs of illness four years after the exposure. Adverse neurological effects have also been reported in association with the phenoxy herbicides, arsenicals, methyl bromide, and rodenticides containing thallium (Abou-Donia & Preissig, 1976a, 1976b; Xintaras et al., 1978). The organophosphorus compounds, in addition to producing acute neurological effects, have also been shown to be associated with intermediate and delayed neurological and psychological effects (Savage et al., 1988). Subtle behavioural changes have been noted in several cross-sectional epidemiological studies among pest control workers, farmers, and manufacturing workers, and behavioural impairments have also been associated with pesticide exposure in serious accidents among agricultural workers (Maizlish et al., 1987; Eskenazi & Maizlish, 1988).

Enzyme induction

Induction of liver microsomal enzymes by pesticides was first demonstrated in animals. In 1969, antipyrine was shown to have a shortened half-life in workers exposed to a variety of pesticides, including primarily DDT, lindane, and chlordane (Kolmodin et al., 1969). Additional confirmation of increased antipyrine metabolism was provided by Guzelian et al. (1980) for organochlorines, and by Dossing (1984) for phenoxyacids, chlorophenols, and other pesticides. Moreover, Hunter et al. (1971) demonstrated increased D-glutaric acid metabolism among workers manufacturing aldrin, dieldrin, or endrin and Guzelian et al. (1980) showed the same change in chlordecone workers.

Effects on immune status

Several investigations have identified possible associations between exposure to pesticides and immune status. For example, Wysocki et al. (1985) compared serum concentrations of IgA, IgM, IgG, and C-3 complement levels among 51 men with occupational exposure to chlorinated pesticides and 28 controls. IgG was increased, while IgM and C-3 were lower among the exposed workers.

Skin effects

Contact dermatitis and allergic sensitization (which also have acute components) have been frequently observed in pesticide workers (Adams, 1983) after exposure to several pesticides, including barban, benomyl, captafol, DDT, lindane, malathion, paraquat, and zineb. Photoallergic reactions have been reported after exposure to hexachlorobenzene, benomyl, and zineb.

Non-occupational exposure

Acute effects

Accidents resulting from unsafe packing and leakage of pesticides during storage or transport may involve large numbers of people. On a number of occasions food has been contaminated in this way. Parathion and endrin have been involved most frequently in such accidents.

The commonest cases of accidental poisoning by pesticides are those in which grain dressed with pesticides has been eaten (Table 19). For instance, in 1971–72 over 6000 people were admitted to hospitals in Iraq with symptoms of food poisoning and more than 400 died, after eating bread that had been prepared from cereals treated with a methylmercury fungicide (WHO, 1976).

Table 19. Episodes of mass poisoning following the consumption of food contaminated with pesticide[a]

Pesticide involved	Contaminated food	Source or type of contamination	Number of cases	Number of deaths	Location and year
Alkylmercury	bread	treated seed grain	200	70	Iraq, 1956
Alkylmercury	bread	treated seed grain	45	20	Guatemala, 1965–1966
Alkylmercury	seed maize		144	20	Ghana, 1967
Ethylmercury	?	treated seed grain	321	35	Iraq, 1961
Methylmercury	flour	treated seed grain	6530	459	Iraq, 1971
Hexachlorobenzene	?	treated seed grain	3000	400	Turkey, 1960–1963
Endrin	flour	spillage during transport or storage	159	0	United Kingdom, 1956
Endrin	flour	spillage during transport or storage	691	24	Qatar, 1967–1970
Endrin	flour	spillage during transport or storage	183	2	Saudi Arabia, 1967
Parathion	wheat?	spillage during transport or storage	360	102	India, 1958
Parathion	flour	spillage during transport or storage	200	8	Egypt, 1958
Parathion	flour	spillage during transport or storage	600	88	Colombia, 1967–1968
Parathion	flour and sugar?	spillage during transport or storage	559	16	Mexico, 1968
Aldicarb	watermelon	not identified	1350	80	USA, 1985
Total			14342	1324	

[a] Sources: Hayes, 1975; Knapp, 1982; Silano, 1985; Green et al., 1987.

Other accidents have occurred when insecticides that have been found to be effective against one type of pest have been incorrectly and dangerously used against other pests, such as bedbugs or body lice, and have resulted in poisoning. In the tropics, containers that have held pesticide concentrates are attractive for household use, but might well cause poisoning if used for carrying water or for cooking food. It is not uncommon for children to drink pesticide solutions if they are not adequately stored. Aerial spraying and drifting have also caused clinical effects in people in nearby areas.

Despite clear warnings on labels, improper use of pesticides has resulted in serious outbreaks of poisoning. For example, pentachlorophenol was used as a terminal rinse for laundering infant diapers despite a warning on the label prohibiting this use (Robson et al., 1969); twenty cases of poisoning resulted, including two deaths. More recently, 1350 cases and eight deaths occurred in California among people who consumed watermelons that had been treated with aldicarb, a systemic pesticide not registered for such use (Green et al., 1987).

Table 19 shows the health impact (numbers of cases and deaths) of accidental exposure to pesticides as a result of eating contaminated food. In some cases, the food was contaminated during transport or storage, in other cases, seeds were consumed that had been treated with fungicides and were intended for planting.

These outbreaks of mass poisoning often affect all age groups. It is important to note that cases of poisoning in children, as a result of accidental exposure to pesticide kept in the home, may occur on a large scale, but often go unidentified unless specific surveys are carried out. The available national mortality statistics indicate that death by poisoning among young children is more common in many developing countries than in developed countries (WHO, 1986e). Pesticides are an important cause of these cases of poisoning, particularly in rural areas (Polchenko et al., 1975).

It should be emphasized that the victims of pesticide poisoning accidents are often members of the general population. In the recent catastrophe in Bhopal, India (where there was an accidental release of toxic raw materials from a pesticide manufacturing plant), for example, most of the casualties were people who lived close to the manufacturing plant.

57

Chronic effects

Cancer

Evaluations by the International Agency for Research on Cancer (pages 37–41 and 53) have been based on occupational exposure and effect data. A recent review of the cancer risks associated with pesticides in agricultural workers (CSA, 1988) included several studies of farmers, which in rural areas in some countries may include the majority of the population in the age range 20–60 years; however, these people are likely to have been exposed to pesticides from several different sources. It should be pointed out that studies of any link between pesticides and cancer in the general population are difficult because generally the exposures are low, the risks are low, and there are opportunities for misclassification of exposure. These factors tend to reduce the likelihood of showing a statistically significant effect, even when there is a known risk. Recent calculations of the potential number of cancer cases in the USA due to pesticide exposure (NAS, 1987) are based on extrapolations from animal data and are highly uncertain (see page 88).

Reproductive effects

It has been suspected (WHO, 1984a) that exposure of men to phenoxyacid herbicides (e.g., "agent Orange") is associated with an increased risk of abortions and malformations in their offspring. A similar association has also been suspected for general population exposure to chlorinated hydrocarbons (WHO, 1979), but so far no satisfactory investigation has been carried out. The question remains of interest however, in view of the estrogenic activity of these agents and their widespread use in developing countries.

Immunological effects

Studies have been carried out in four geographical areas in Moldavia, USSR; three of these had different levels of environmental pesticide burden, and one had a low level of pesticide use (Kozlyuk et al., 1987). Associations were found between the amount of pesticide used in the area and both the occurrence of immunological imbalance and the incidence of infectious diseases in children.

Respiratory effects

Some cases of asthma have been reported to be linked to exposure to organophosphorus pesticides (Hayes, 1982), but it is uncertain whether it was the active ingredient or another component in the formulation that produced the effects. The possibility has been studied that paraquat may have been the cause of chronic fibrotic changes seen in the survivors of suicide attempts (WHO, 1984c).

Ophthalmological and neuro-ophthalmological effects

Optic nerve atrophy has been noted in case reports following exposure to methyl bromide (Chavez et al., 1985). Misra et al. (1985) found macular changes in 19% of 79 subjects exposed to the organophosphorus pesticide fenthion, as compared with 3 of 100 controls. Differences in age, height, weight, alcohol intake, smoking, and energy intake did not appear to account for the observed effects. The average age of subjects with macular involvement was 30.6 years and their average duration of pesticide exposure was 7.9 years. The symptoms reported included dislike of bright light, black dots in front of the eyes, and visual blurring. However, 53% of the workers with macular changes did not have ocular symptoms.

Pesticides that deserve to be given priority in future studies

In view of the lack of knowledge on the health effects of pesticides, many more studies are required and these should concentrate on compounds that are used extensively and that produce recognized effects or effects that are suspected on the basis of animal experiments or *in vitro* tests.

A limited number of pesticides deserve priority for further studies (Table 18). All of them can produce severe effects on human health or the environment, and their use has consequently been severely restricted or banned in many developed countries and in certain developing countries. They are, however, still used extensively in other developing countries. Data on the estimated annual production of these pesticides in different countries are given in Annex 1.

The organochlorine insecticides aldrin, dieldrin, endrin, camphechlor, chlordane, heptachlor, HCH, lindane, DDT, and mirex are persistent, fat-soluble substances that accumulate in the food chain. These substances and some of their metabolites have been found in human fatty tissues and human milk in countries all over the world. Aldrin, dieldrin, and endrin have the highest acute toxicity in this group of pesticides. Furthermore, several of these organochlorine insecticides have shown sufficient or limited evidence of carcinogenicity in long-term animal studies. There is increasing evidence that they are active cancer promoters.

The insecticide parathion and the nematocide aldicarb are extremely potent inhibitors of cholinesterase and have been implicated in many unintentional and intentional poisonings and deaths. Substances like parathion and aldicarb are especially hazardous in countries where there is a lack of education and training in the proper handling of pesticides, and a lack of medical facilities.

The International Agency for Research on Cancer considers that ethylene dibromide shows sufficient evidence of carcinogenicity. As it is a fumigant, it is likely that the use of this compound in developing countries with inadequate equipment may lead to hazardous exposure.

The widely used multipurpose herbicide paraquat has been reported as the cause of many cases of severe or fatal intoxication (WHO, 1984c). Many of these poisonings have been intentional. As the intoxication is characterized by delayed effects in the lung with pulmonary fibrosis, the effects of chronic exposure to lower, non-fatal doses cannot be excluded.

Both pentachlorophenol and 2,4,5-trichlorophenoxyacetic acid may be contaminated with highly toxic and carcinogenic polychlorinated dioxins and dibenzofurans during production, and thus constitute a possible long-term threat to human health.

Chapter 5

SOURCES AND INDICATORS OF HUMAN EXPOSURE TO PESTICIDES

Human exposure to pesticides can be described in several ways, e.g., acute or chronic, occupational or non-occupational, intentional or unintentional, accidental or incidental. Within each type the exposure can be oral (by mouth), respiratory (by inhalation), or dermal (through the skin). The different categories of exposure were depicted in Fig. 1. Since individuals are often exposed in more than one way, the total exposure from all sources needs to be considered in assessing the health risk.

The *potential exposure* from the environment can be estimated by environmental monitoring. The *actual exposure* (uptake) can be measured by biological monitoring of human tissues and body fluids.

Acute exposure

Acute exposures may be accidental, occupational, or intentional and may lead to either systemic effects or local effects (such as dermatitis or lesions in the eye). Apart from poisonings in the home environment, systemic poisoning is found in workers, and the exposure is predominantly dermal, with contaminated clothing being especially important. Inhalation is the second most common route of acute exposure for workers producing or using agricultural chemicals. For the general public, however, ingestion—either accidental or intentional—is the most common route of exposure. Both adults and children are at risk of poisoning, storage in improper containers being a common causal factor in acute exposure in children.

Accidental exposure

Overall, accidental exposure to pesticides accounts for about 4–5% of all accidental poisonings; this proportion is higher in developing countries than in industrialized countries. Drugs and household poisons are much more likely to be the agents involved, but one must remember that these chemicals are more likely to be readily available in a much larger number of households than are pesticides. The chief victims of acute accidental exposure to pesticides are children under five years of age.

Owing to the very high toxicity of some of the commonly used pesticides, the ingestion of even very small amounts (1 g or less), or limited skin contact with the concentrated product, can lead to acute poisoning. Some examples of situations where non-occupational, accidental exposure to pesticides needs to be considered are the following:

— pesticides stored in unlocked cabinets in a dwelling (accessible to children);

— pesticides stored in unmarked bottles or containers, which may be swallowed in mistake for food or drink;

— storage of pesticides close to bulk foodstuffs;

— use of farm pesticides for household or medical purposes, when extensive skin contact or inhalation may arise;

— use of empty pesticide containers to transport or store drinking-water;

— treatment of foodstuffs with pesticides or treatment of seed grains with fungicides;

— transport of food and pesticides in the same lorry or in the same part of a ship.

The last two of these situations are of particular concern, because one incident of food contamination or misuse of treated seed grains can affect large populations, such as happened in Iraq in 1970 (see Chapter 4). Several severe poisoning incidents have occurred as a result of this type of exposure (Table 19). Still the general impression of the extent of ill health caused by accidental contamination of food by pesticides (excluding the metal- and metalloid-based fungicides) is that major incidents are rare, in relation to the widespread use of these chemicals. Hayes (1975), in his standard work on the health hazards of pesticides, cited 28 major outbreaks of pesticide poisoning due to contaminated food over a period of 40 years. There appears to have been a reduction in the last decade compared with previous decades.

Occupational exposure

About 60–70% of all cases of unintentional acute pesticide poisoning are due to occupational exposure (Copplestone, 1985) and workers in developing countries appear to be at particular risk. When pesticides are used in agriculture, the occupational groups that may be exposed include farmers and members of farming families. It is not uncommon for a whole family, including children and elderly family members, to be involved in the work on a farm, particularly in developing countries. When estimating the number of people at risk from acute occupational exposure, this has to be taken into account.

Occupational exposure may also occur among people involved in the manufacture and processing of pesticides. In addition, pesticide residues on plants or fruits may cause significant exposure in farmworkers picking or handling the produce. The following list shows some of the occupations with potential exposure in these industries:

— pesticide manufacturers (production workers)
— formulators
— vendors
— transporters
— mixers
— loaders
— operators of application equipment (farmers or professionals)
— growers and pickers
— rescue and clean-up parties.

Intentional exposure

People may expose themselves to pesticides intentionally in an attempt to commit suicide. The main route of exposure is ingestion. This is likely to represent a significant problem whenever pesticides with high toxicity are freely available in the community. The easy availability of chemicals that kill quickly so that there is no time for rescue (e.g., parathion), or kill after a delay during which treatment is ineffective (e.g., paraquat), increases the occurrence of fatal intentional exposures.

Long-term occupational exposure

Long-term occupational exposure is likely to occur in the occupational groups listed above. Very few reports of such effects are available and further studies are needed to investigate the conditions under which chronic exposure does occur. For instance, long-term exposure in working environments with high levels of pesticide dust may eventually lead to chronic effects in the lungs, even if no acute poisoning occurs. Chronic exposure to a pesticide that can cause cancer in animals should be recorded, even if the exposure is considered low, so that any possible link with human cancer can be detected. Chronic exposure of workers to some pesticides can be measured by biological monitoring (see p. 69), which provides the most reliable estimates of the long-term uptake of the chemical in the body.

Long-term exposure in the general environment

The general population may be exposed to pesticides in several ways. The main routes of exposure are listed below in order of importance:

1. ingestion (via food and drinking-water),
2. inhalation (via air and dust), and
3. skin absorption (via clothing or direct contact).

Residents living in, or close to, farming areas, may be exposed to pesticide sprays in the air, depending on their proximity to the crops being treated, and in contaminated water or food. Consumers far away from farming areas may eat crops or animal products, or drink water, contaminated with pesticide residues. In addition, there may be exposure via air, water, and food, as a result of the use of pesticides in public health programmes to kill disease vectors in residential areas.

Air

Air can easily become contaminated with pesticides during spraying operations. The evaporation of droplets during the spraying of emulsified formulations may result in the formation of tiny particles that can be carried great distances in air currents. This has been confirmed, for example, by studies showing the presence of pesticides in urban smog (Glotfelty et al., 1987).

It has been shown that even relatively non-volatile pesticides, such as DDT, evaporate into the atmosphere quite rapidly, particularly in hot climates, when pesticides are desorbed from the clay and organic fractions in soil. In the tropics, about 90% of organochlorine insecticides in the soil may disappear in one year. Other pesticides can volatilize even more rapidly. Even herbicides with a low vapour pressure (e.g., 2,4-D esters) are volatilized, especially during spraying operations.

However, according to Edwards (1986), there is little evidence of any serious effects of exposure to airborne pesticides on human health, except where pesticides are used in enclosed and unventilated spaces.

It is a common practice in many developing countries to treat human habitations with pesticides to control disease vectors. The chemical evaporates into the air in the house and may be inhaled by the inhabitants. Further amounts may be taken through the skin by contact with treated surfaces, or ingested with contaminated food.

There is evidence from India of cows taking up organo-chlorine insecticides by rubbing against treated walls, following which significant amounts of the pesticides appeared in the cows' milk (Edwards et al., 1980).

Soil

Soil may be deliberately treated with pesticides to control insects, nematodes, or diseases. In addition, it has been calculated that as much as 50% of the pesticide sprayed on crops or used as a herbicide misses its target and falls on to the soil surface. Some pesticides, notably organochlorines, may persist in soil for years (Edwards, 1986), even though, as mentioned above, a large proportion evaporates.

The persistence and transport of pesticides in soils depend on several factors such as the chemical structure of the com-pound, type of formulation, type of soil, weather conditions, irrigation, type of crop, and the microorganisms present in the soil.

Pesticides may be taken up from the soil by crops, especially root vegetables, such as carrots. If grass is grown, the residues in the grass may be ingested by herbivores such as cattle, and eventually find their way into meat and milk. Fortunately, some pesticides become adsorbed on clay particles and organic matter in soils in a form which is not readily taken up by plants. There is still, however, a danger of their polluting groundwater supplies.

According to Edwards (1986), there is little evidence that pesticide contamination of soils has serious effects on human health, because the amounts taken up by crops are small, and result in little food contamination. However, in one recent outbreak of poisoning due to contamination of watermelons by aldicarb (Green et al., 1987), one possible explanation of the contamination was uptake of the pesticide from the soil.

Water

Many human disease vectors are controlled through the spraying or treating of surface water with insecticides. Herbicides are often applied to water in tropical areas to control aquatic weeds. In addition, water may be polluted by:

— discharges of surplus pesticide, after spraying operations;

— water used for washing spraying equipment being poured into rivers, ponds, or lakes;

— crops to be sprayed being planted right up to the water's edge;

— accidental spillage of pesticide formulations;

— run-off, leakage, and erosion from treated soils;

— fall-out of pesticides from polluted air;

— application of pesticides to rivers or ponds, to kill fish, which are then removed and eaten.

Any of these routes may lead to contamination of drinking-water. Nevertheless, average exposure to pesticides from drinking-water is generally low, although serious incidents do occur occasionally (Edwards, 1986).

Measurements of levels of organochlorine pesticides in drinking-water sources have been carried out as part of the UNEP/WHO Global Environmental Monitoring System (GEMS, 1983). The drinking-water guideline values published by WHO (1984f) were exceeded in rivers in five countries and in lakes in three countries. The highest value was 1000 times the guideline value. Estimates of the corresponding human exposures were not made. More of the data collected by GEMS have since been published by UNEP/WHO (1987, 1988).

Crops

The concentration of pesticide on a crop directly after spraying needs to be high enough to be effective against the pest. The ratio between the effective concentration and the concentration that will affect human health if the crop is consumed is of major importance in assessing the hazard associated with exposure.

Pesticides on crops will evaporate, be washed off, break down, or become absorbed into the plant material. The concentration also drops as a result of dilution as the plant grows. Because the concentration of the pesticide in and on the crop decreases, a pesticide application that was initially very toxic to human subjects may with time become harmless. For this reason, farmers are advised not to spray just before harvest, and in many developed countries, the "waiting periods" are formally established and part of good agricultural practice.

The exposure of the general population to pesticides that have been applied to crops correctly according to good agricultural practice has been assessed by WHO and FAO, and reported in a series of data sheets on more than 70 individual pesticides (WHO/FAO, 1975–1989). For all the pesticides reviewed, it was concluded that good agricultural practice does not result in exposure to hazardous amounts.

Because it is desirable to lose as little as possible of the yield of crops intended for human consumption, in general more pesticides are applied to them than to other less valuable crops. Moreover, in developing countries there is usually little control or advice on the timing of the applications; often pesticides are applied only days or hours before the crops are harvested. Such crops may contain residues that lead to high exposures if the crops are consumed soon after harvest. In some countries, this is a major problem because many vegetables are grown on small plots close to towns and the treated crops go straight to the market, often with little washing. Sometimes they may even be treated with pesticides in the marketplace to control flies. Such misuse of pesticides must be stopped.

Food

Apart from direct contamination caused by spraying, there are various other ways in which foodstuffs can be contaminated. For example, meat may contain high levels of pesticides because they become concentrated in certain tissues, following cattle dipping or vector treatment. Fish caught in pesticide-treated rice paddies may also contain significant levels of pesticide residues.

Treatment with pesticides to prevent losses of food during storage or bulk transport also creates a hazard (UNEP, 1981). The losses caused by arthropod pests and rodents can be extremely heavy and it is a common practice to treat food and grain with pesticides, more or less indiscriminately, to avoid such losses. Food treated in this way may contain high concentrations of pesticide.

In times of shortage, there have been many instances of pesticide-treated seed grains being eaten by people or domestic animals, either accidentally or intentionally and producing mass poisoning. Cooking or processing a contaminated foodstuff may modify the toxicity of the pesticide, and this fact should be considered in epidemiological studies of food exposure to pesticides.

Many countries have legislation relating to food contamination, and imported and local foods are regularly analysed. In some developing countries, however, there is little legislation, pest problems are often much greater, and spraying close to harvest is common because of lack of knowledge (Edwards, 1986).

The development of international standards to avoid excessive food contamination has been the main purpose of the Joint FAO/WHO Food Standards Programme and the Codex Alimentarius Commission (Codex, 1984).

Data on pesticide residues in foodstuffs are available from a variety of sources, ranging from precise studies using radio-labelled materials, through supervised trials in different agricultural and climatic conditions, to commodity monitoring when the treatment history of the sample is unknown. It is important to recognize the limitations of each type of study (Bates, 1982). However, when specific data are available on pesticide use and on the residues in food in the same area, a direct correlation can sometimes be demonstrated (Kapoor et al., 1980).

In 1979, the UNEP/FAO/WHO Collaborating Centres for Food Contamination Monitoring were asked to submit all available data on the levels of certain chemical contaminants in the total diet and to provide details on how the total dietary intakes were determined. Since 1980, these data have been collected systematically within the framework of the UNEP/WHO Global Environmental Monitoring System (GEMS, 1986).

Data on certain pesticides were received from eleven collaborating centres participating in the monitoring programme in Australia, Austria, Canada, Guatemala, Hungary, Ireland, Japan, New Zealand, Sweden, the United Kingdom, and the United States of America. The data cover the period from 1971 to 1983 and include information on the intakes of several organochlorine and organophosphorus pesticides (Table 20). In order to identify potential health problems possibly associated with the presence of toxic contaminants in the food supply, an analysis was made of actual dietary intakes of certain contaminants. In some cases, the intakes of aldrin, dieldrin, and lindane reached levels close to the ADI established by the joint FAO/WHO Meetings on Pesticide Residues.

Biological monitoring

Human exposure to pesticides is usually estimated by measuring levels in the environment (air, water, and food). In some cases, however, information on exposure can be obtained by analysis of the concentrations of the specific pesticides in human body tissues and fluids. This is termed biological monitoring and is particularly useful when there is simultaneous exposure via several routes. Biological monitoring requires special staff and facilities to collect and analyse the samples, and to interpret the results. Consequently, this approach has been used only to a limited extent in developing countries.

UNEP and WHO have carried out several projects within the framework of GEMS to encourage the application of biological monitoring in countries and to improve the available methods. A pilot project incorporating both environmental and biological monitoring (GEMS Human Exposure Assessment Location Programme, HEAL) is in progress at present.

Indicators of exposure

Incidental exposures to several persistent and non-persistent pesticides and their metabolites, can be determined by analysis of serum, fat, urine, blood, or breast milk (Table 21). For

Table 20. Summary of GEMS dietary intake studies of organochlorine and organophosphorus pesticides[a]

Pesticide	Maximum ADI (mg/kg of body weight)	Summary of results	Assessment
Aldrin and dieldrin	0.0001 (combined total aldrin + dieldrin) (1966)	Median and/or mean dietary intakes of aldrin/dieldrin residues reported by several countries represent a significant percentage of the ADI. In the most recent years, median values range from 5% to 15% of the ADI while mean values range from 7% to 56% of the ADI. In one case, the 90th percentile exceeded the ADI. A decrease in dietary intake of residues of aldrin/dieldrin over a period of years has occurred in some countries. This may be due to the introduction by some countries of restrictions or bans on the use of these pesticides.	All the reported 90th percentile values were below the residue limits established for the foods monitored. The 90th percentile levels of aldrin and dieldrin in human milk were above those in cow's milk, but were below the ERL[b] of 150 µg/kg (fat basis) for cow's milk.
DDT complex	0.02 (1984)	The dietary intakes of the DDT complex were low in the reporting countries. All 90th percentile values were below 10% of the ADI.	With the exception of the level of DDT complex in lettuce from one part of Egypt, none of the median or 90th percentile levels submitted were above the Codex residue limits. A comparatively high 90th percentile level of DDT complex in tomatoes was reported in Australia. The participating countries submitted very few data on the DDT complex in raw commodities. Thus, it is difficult to assess the likelihood of DDT contamination of these products, especially in developing countries where it is or has been used more extensively. The 90th percentile levels for DDT in human milk from all reporting countries were above the Codex limit for DDT in cow's milk. The levels reported by Guatemala were lower than those reported previously, but both the median and 90th percentile levels were appreciably above the Codex limit.

Levels of DDT and other chlorinated pesticides in human milk should be monitored more frequently and by more countries. There is also a need to identify the sources of contamination and to evaluate the possible health implications of the levels found.

Hexachloro-cyclohexanes (HCH), total isomers	0.01 (gamma-isomer (lindane)) (1977)	No ADI has been proposed by the Joint FAO/WHO Meeting on Pesticide Residues for total HCH isomers. In Canada, the intake of hexachlorocyclohexane (HCH) isomers decreased from 0.05 μg/kg of body weight in 1971 to 0.01 μg/kg of body weight in 1977. The median intakes reported by Guatemala, Japan, and the United Kingdom were generally around 0.4 μg/kg of body weight. Hungary reported intakes of various population groups. The overall median values were 0.2 and 0.1 μg/kg of body weight in 1978 and 1979 respectively. In the USA, mean intakes showed an increase from 0.004 to 0.025 μg/kg of body weight between 1972 and 1974, at which point a decreasing trend is noticeable down to a value of 0.01 μg/kg of body weight in 1982.	Overall, low levels of total HCH isomers were found in the food supply, with no evidence of an increase since 1979. Consistent with this is the fact that the levels in human milk appear to be remaining steady, or perhaps decreasing slowly. However, the levels in human milk are higher than in cow's milk in countries where a comparison can be made (Japan, United Kingdom, USA). High levels of total HCH isomers were found in milk and dairy products in certain countries where this pesticide may have been used more recently. It is also of interest that lower levels have been reported in milk from Canada, the United Kingdom and the USA than elsewhere.

High levels of total HCH isomers reported from the United Kingdom in imported pork fat and to a lesser extent in domestic hen fat indicate that sporadic incidents of contamination of food of animal origin may occur as a result of the presence of HCH in the environment.

Comparatively high levels of total HCH in maize and rice from China are an indication that residues of this pesticide do occur in foods of vegetable origin, probably as a result of recent usage. In view of the concern about technical grade HCH, its occurrence in domestic and imported foods and in human milk warrants increased control of its use and monitoring for its residues in the food supply.

71

Table 20 (continued)

Pesticide	Maximum ADI (mg/kg of body weight)	Summary of results	Assessment
Lindane	0.01 (1977)	Dietary intake data on lindane residues were submitted by Guatemala, Japan, New Zealand, the United Kingdom, and the USA. All intakes reported constituted 1.2% or less of the ADI, even at the 90th percentile levels.	Generally, the levels of lindane in most foods, with the exception of milk and fresh produce, were well below Codex limits. For milk, the 90th percentile levels in some cases approached the Codex residue limit. There also was some indication of a contamination incident involving milk in one year in the United Kingdom. These results indicate that continued monitoring for lindane in milk and in cattle feed is called for. Levels reported for lindane residue in other foods were generally low. One exception was high levels of lindane in fresh produce, probably resulting from recent and extensive use.
Heptachlor/ heptachlor epoxide	0.0005 (1966)	Dietary intakes of heptachlor and heptachlor epoxide residues have been reported by Canada, Guatemala, Japan, and the USA. In every case, the median intakes were 1% or less of the ADI of 0.5 μg/kg of body weight. The highest 90th percentile intakes reported were 9% and 3% of the ADI in Guatemala and Japan, respectively, in 1982.	There is little evidence of contamination of foods by heptachlor, HCB or endosulfan, except for milk and human milk. However, the elevated levels of HCB, and to a lesser extent, heptachlor plus its epoxide in human milk as compared to cow's milk indicate the continued need to reduce sources of contamination by these pesticides.
Hexachloro-benzene (HCB)	ADI (=0.0006) withdrawn 1978	No significant trend is apparent in countries reporting data for several years (Canada, Japan, and the USA). The median intake of HCB in 1973–77 varied from 0.001 to 0.13 μg/kg of body weight in the diets studied in Canada, Hungary, Japan, United Kingdom, and the USA. More recently, the median dietary intakes of HCB were	In addition, the evidence of an incident of fish contamination by HCB (Brazil reported median and 90th percentile levels of 30 μg/kg and 200 μg/kg, respectively, in canned fish from one part of the country in 1983) also indicates the continued need to reduce sources of contamination and to monitor for these pesticides in food of animal origin.
Endosulfan	0.008 (1982)	reported to be in the vicinity of 0.002 μg/kg of body weight, with no significant differences between the different countries.	

| Organo-phosphorus pesticides | Diazinon: 0.002 (1965)
Malathion: 0.02 (1963)
Parathion: 0.005 (1963)
Parathion-methyl: 0.02 (1984)
Fenitrothion: 0.003 (1986) | For endosulfan, very few samples showed levels above the detection limit; no estimates of dietary intake were made

Collection of dietary intake data on diazinon, malathion, parathion, and parathion-methyl was initiated in 1980. In all cases the median and 90th percentile intake reported for organophosphorus pesticides were low, 2% (or less) of the ADI for the pesticide concerned. For countries reporting data over several years (Japan and the USA), a slight increase in intake of organophosphorus pesticides is seen in more recent years. It will be necessary to obtain data for additional years to determine whether this constitutes a trend. Guatemala reported non-detectable levels for three of the organophosphorus pesticides: malathion, parathion, and parathion-methyl. | Data suggest that when diazinon is applied properly, the levels remaining on the produce when it reaches the market will be very low, near the limit of detection. However, the few exceptions indicate that when the pesticide is misused the levels of residues can approach the MRL.
The data reported so far do not indicate any general occurrence of significant levels of malathion in the foods examined. The 90th percentile levels in wheat indicate the need for continued monitoring specially in grains.
The data reported so far on levels of parathion indicate that it does not occur substantially above the detection limits in most cases. However, sporadic instances of higher levels in fruit and vegetables indicate that contamination of crops can occur under certain conditions of use.
Generally, parathion-methyl was not detected in the foods analysed. However, its occurrence in vegetables in one country in one year at levels above the MRL indicates that contamination at levels of concern can occur under certain conditions of use.
No findings of residues of fenitrothion were reported in the monitoring carried out in 1982 and 1983. However, no assessment can be made until data on residues of this pesticide in foods are reported for a longer period of time and by a greater number of countries. |

[a] Source: GEMS, 1986.

[b] Extraneous residue limit: the maximum toxicologically acceptable concentration of a residue arising from sources other than the use of a pesticide directly or indirectly for the production of the commodity (FAO/WHO (1976)).

Table 21. Biological indicators of exposure to pesticides[a]

Indicator	Uses
Urinary residues of pesticides and their metabolites	Verification of short-term, long-term, and incidental exposure to organophosphorus and carbamate insecticides, phenoxyacid herbicides, paraquat, pentachlorophenol, and others
Adipose and serum residues of pesticides	Verification of short-term, long-term, and incidental exposure to organochlorine and certain lipophilic organophosphorus pesticides
Breast milk residues of pesticides	Verification of short-term and long-term exposure to organochlorine pesticides
Skin and hair residues	Verification of exposure to trace metals (mercury, arsenic)
Cholinesterase determinations	Verification of cholinergic illness and monitoring of exposure to organophosphorus insecticides
Increased blood coagulation time	Indication of exposure to anticoagulant rodenticides

[a] Source: Davies et al., 1982. Reproduced by kind permission of the publisher.

organophosphorus pesticides, cholinesterase activity may be used as an indicator of exposure, since there is a good correlation between exposure and cholinesterase reduction.

Studies have shown that many of the persistent organochlorine pesticides can be found in human fat. The reported levels vary among countries (Table 22), the highest levels of DDT being found in countries where the compound is still used. A detailed review of available data has been published (Murakami, 1987).

Residues in human milk

The first recognition that human milk may be contaminated with environmental chemicals came in 1951, when Laug et al. showed that milk from healthy women in the USA contained considerable amounts of the organochlorine insecticide, DDT. Since then, many investigations of the contamination of human milk have been made in countries all over the world, and DDT and some other organochlorine pesticides have been detected in most of these investigations. The contaminants found most frequently in human milk have been DDT, its main metabolite DDE, hexachlorobenzene, hexachlorocyclohexane, dieldrin, heptachlor epoxide, and the non-pesticide polychlorinated biphenyls.

Table 22. Organochlorine insecticides found in human
fat in the general population of different
countries before the restriction or ban of
organochlorine insecticides in the developed
countries

Country	Insecticide	Amount (mg/kg)
Argentina	total DDT	13.2
	beta-HCH	2.4
	dieldrin	0.3
	heptachlor epoxide	0.2
Brazil	total DDT	7.9
	beta-HCH	0.2
	dieldrin	0.1
	heptachlor epoxide	0.002
Canada	total DDT	4.9
France	total DDT	7.1
	HCH	0.1
	heptachlor epoxide	0.1
India	total DDT	31.0
	dieldrin	0.03
United Kingdom	total DDT	3.0
	HCH	0.3
	dieldrin	0.2
USA	total DDT	9.6
	HCH	0.5
	dieldrin	0.1

[a] Source: W. F. Almeida, personal communication.

In a recent Swedish study of human milk (Norén, 1987), the
levels of polychlorinated dioxins and dibenzofurans (PCDs and
PCDFs) were found to have declined during the 10 previous
years. It was suggested that the decline was at least partly due
to the prohibition in Sweden of the use of certain pesticides
such as chlorinated phenols and 2,4,5-T. All these pesticides
contain various amounts of the highly toxic PCDs and PCDFs
as contaminants.

Data on pesticide residues in human milk have recently been
collected and evaluated in the Joint FAO/WHO Food
Contamination Monitoring Programme. A summary of the
data and estimations of intake for certain pesticides are given
in Table 23.

The dietary intake of contaminants by breast-fed infants may
be estimated from the residue levels found in human milk. For
the first three months of life, an infant consumes on average

Table 23. GEMS estimates of intake of selected pesticides from human milk[a]

Pesticide	Estimated intake
aldrin and dieldrin	Data from 11 countries indicate that, in all cases, the 90th percentile exceeds the maximum ADI of 0.1 µg/kg of body weight by up to ten times. Most median values also exceed the ADI
DDT complex	On the basis of an "acceptable level" for DDT in milk (see text) of 167 µg/kg, the ADI was exceeded at the 90th percentile level in recent years only in Guatemala. The 90th percentile intake amounted to approximately 70% of the ADI in the USA in 1979
lindane	Data submitted on median and 90th percentile levels of lindane in human milk indicate that in all cases the estimated intakes were well below the maximum ADI of 10 µg/kg of body weight, never exceeding 10% of the ADI even at the 90th percentile level
heptachlor and heptachlor epoxide	At the 90th percentile level, the calculated intake at times constituted an appreciable percentage of the ADI; in the USA (1975 and 1979) and Switzerland (1974) this calculated intake amounted to approximately 85% of the ADI. Calculated 90th percentile intakes in Guatemala (1974) and Japan (1978) were at approximately the 75% level, but decreased in subsequent years

[a] Source: GEMS, 1986

120 g of human milk per kg of body weight per day, the volume consumed per unit weight decreasing with increasing age. By multiplying the concentration of a given contaminant in µg/kg by 0.12, the approximate intake of the contaminant may be estimated in µg/kg of body weight per day; this may be compared with the relevant ADI. Alternatively, an "acceptable level" of a pesticide residue in human milk may be computed by dividing the ADI by 0.12. For example, the maximum "acceptable level" of aldrin/dieldrin in human milk is 0.8 µg/kg (whole milk) (based on an ADI of 0–0.0001 mg/kg of body weight); at concentrations of aldrin/dieldrin greater than 0.8 µg/kg of whole milk a breast-fed infant would take in more than the ADI.

However, as pointed out by a recent expert group (WHO, 1987b), an ADI can be misleading for infants when it concerns compounds that accumulate in fatty tissues. Owing to the rapid increase in fat during the first 6 months of life, even a comparatively high intake of a fat-soluble compound might not lead to a correspondingly high concentration of the compound at the target sites.

The expert group concluded that there is no justification at present for limiting breast-feeding or for eliminating specific food items from the mother's diet. Despite the presence of these compounds in human milk, breast-feeding should be encouraged and promoted because of the benefits of mother's milk to the overall health and development of the infant. However, in population groups in which this type of pesticide contamination is a problem, active intervention to reduce the contamination is essential.

Factors influencing exposure

There have been many advances in developed countries in methods of application of pesticides, with the use of seed dressings, precise spot treatments, smaller and smaller quantities of spray, and methods involving ultra-low-volume (ULV) sprays. Consequently, application has become progressively safer. Closed systems, in which the plants are enclosed in a greenhouse-type structure while being sprayed, offer the possibility of markedly reducing exposure; however, without proper maintenance, they may lead to a false sense of security. In contrast, much of the application equipment used in developing countries is poorly maintained and supplies of spares are inadequate. Pesticides are often applied with inefficient hand-sprayers, ox-drawn sprayers, or dusting equipment, and inadequate protective clothing is used. In addition, in many developing countries, the hot climatic conditions and the general lack of education make pesticide use more dangerous to the operator than in developed countries.

In the developed countries, much of the pesticide used is applied by professional operators. In developing countries, pesticides are applied almost entirely by farmers, many of whom have insufficient education and training in the different methods of application. The farmers often lack awareness of the potential hazards and do not take elementary precautions. For this reason, an effective network of extension and advisory services, which provide technical advice on the safe use of pesticides, can be of great value in preventing health effects. Many developing countries have no extension service and advice comes mainly from representatives of pesticide manufacturers. Pesticides are often applied at too frequent intervals, particularly when they are first used in a country, at which time the yields increase dramatically.

systems

and thus the possible
farming systems. In
cater for local needs
in this type of agri-
ted" or controlled in
ited, as the farmers
r cannot afford them,

agriculture, some
ands of the subsistence
tential risks and

eveloping countries is
on for the regional,
own in Table 7 (page
is in the production
s, rice, corn and

can be categorized in
onditions, method of
of commercialization.
defined by
are: plantation farming,
uires intensive pest
in both the types of
; and subsistence
n important role in
nd the more the crop
hood that pesticides
influence, the two
eing cotton and rice.
n all types of agri-
can be controlled by

human effort, although Papua New Guinea is a notable exception (Mowbray, 1988).

In plantations, employees may be provided with housing, food, and some medical care. Plantations vary in the care and training provided and sometimes set their own standards rather than conform to any minimum national standard of working conditions. Pesticide use may be high but the amount of exposure usually depends on the quality of management. Pesticides are often used on a large scale using aircraft or tractor-driven equipment.

On most farms with cash-crops the situation is different in many respects. Many cash-crop farms are family affairs, while on others families, rather than individuals, are employed to carry out the routine operations. Thus, large sections of the rural population are involved. In some developing countries, these people may make up more than half the total rural population, excluding plantation workers and those too old or too young to work in the fields or look after the flocks. In general, the cash-cropping farmers use smaller quantities of pesticides than the plantation farmers, either because of lack of access or because of the high cost.

As pointed out by Copplestone (1985), the likelihood of exposure to pesticides depends on family structure and traditional living habits. Where the farmers and their families live close to the fields the risk of exposure is higher than where they live in villages and walk long distances to their work.

For subsistence farmers, there is much less exposure to pesticides because usually they cannot afford the products. They must suffer the crop losses caused by pests, and probably represent the group least exposed to pesticides (Copplestone, 1985).

The most important crops with respect to pesticide use are cotton, rice, and maize. Certain plantation crops such as fruits, coffee, and tea are also important, but they are grown on much smaller areas. In the developing parts of the world, cotton, rice, and maize are grown on 27, 140, and 80 million hectares, respectively. Coffee plantations make up another 10.5 million hectares. More details are shown in Table 24.

However, only a small part of the rice and maize production can be regarded as pesticide-intensive. Most of these crops are

on authorities require the
ate and safe, to minimize
st, the labelling and
countries are often
area where they are
a language that the user
is explained poorly or
he pesticide are usually not
ecified. Guidelines on
ublished by FAO (1985b).

e is a limited number of
available, in developing
range of formulations of
cally. Unscrupulous
out-of-date ineffective
be noted that the World
e of pesticides in projects
that materials that are
hould be made available
lations. The recommen-
complete protection of
conditions. Water-soluble
nd microencapsulated
gh the last two are, at

propriate protective
eveloping countries many
ring inadequate or unsuit-
ently worn for extensive
pesticides, so increasing
al. Moreover, in hot
lom be used, because the
so high that the worker

eas to spray the walls of
control household pests
os. These pesticides have a
ants are exposed continu-
r by contact or inhalation,
food (Edwards, 1986).

The expert group concluded that there is no justification at present for limiting breast-feeding or for eliminating specific food items from the mother's diet. Despite the presence of these compounds in human milk, breast-feeding should be encouraged and promoted because of the benefits of mother's milk to the overall health and development of the infant. However, in population groups in which this type of pesticide contamination is a problem, active intervention to reduce the contamination is essential.

Factors influencing exposure

There have been many advances in developed countries in methods of application of pesticides, with the use of seed dressings, precise spot treatments, smaller and smaller quantities of spray, and methods involving ultra-low-volume (ULV) sprays. Consequently, application has become progressively safer. Closed systems, in which the plants are enclosed in a greenhouse-type structure while being sprayed, offer the possibility of markedly reducing exposure; however, without proper maintenance, they may lead to a false sense of security. In contrast, much of the application equipment used in developing countries is poorly maintained and supplies of spares are inadequate. Pesticides are often applied with inefficient hand-sprayers, ox-drawn sprayers, or dusting equipment, and inadequate protective clothing is used. In addition, in many developing countries, the hot climatic conditions and the general lack of education make pesticide use more dangerous to the operator than in developed countries.

In the developed countries, much of the pesticide used is applied by professional operators. In developing countries, pesticides are applied almost entirely by farmers, many of whom have insufficient education and training in the different methods of application. The farmers often lack awareness of the potential hazards and do not take elementary precautions. For this reason, an effective network of extension and advisory services, which provide technical advice on the safe use of pesticides, can be of great value in preventing health effects. Many developing countries have no extension service and advice comes mainly from representatives of pesticide manufacturers. Pesticides are often applied at too frequent intervals, particularly when they are first used in a country, at which time the yields increase dramatically.

In developed countries, the registration authorities require the labelling and packaging to be adequate and safe, to minimize excessive or unnecessary use. In contrast, the labelling and packaging of pesticides in developing countries are often inadequate and inappropriate for the area where they are used. The advice is often written in a language that the user does not understand and the toxicity is explained poorly or not at all; the appropriate uses of the pesticide are usually not stated clearly and the dosages not specified. Guidelines on good labelling practices have been published by FAO (1985b).

Whereas in developed countries there is a limited number of types and formulations of pesticides available, in developing countries there may be a bewildering range of formulations of the same chemical, often prepared locally. Unscrupulous formulators may add diluents or use out-of-date ineffective chemicals. In this connection it may be noted that the World Bank (1985), in its guidelines for use of pesticides in projects financed by the Bank, recommended that materials that are likely to become widely distributed should be made available only in relatively low-toxicity formulations. The recommendation is based on the concept that complete protection of workers cannot be expected in hot conditions. Water-soluble packages and free-flowing granular and microencapsulated formulations are safe to use, although the last two are, at present, very expensive.

Even in developed countries, the appropriate protective clothing is often not worn and in developing countries many pesticides are applied by people wearing inadequate or unsuitable clothing. This clothing is frequently worn for extensive periods after being contaminated by pesticides, so increasing the overall exposure of the individual. Moreover, in hot climates, protective clothing can seldom be used, because the temperature inside the clothing gets so high that the worker suffers.

It is common practice in tropical areas to spray the walls of huts and houses with insecticides to control household pests and disease vectors such as mosquitos. These pesticides have a residual action and thus the inhabitants are exposed continually to low levels of pesticides, either by contact or inhalation, and to some extent in contaminated food (Edwards, 1986).

Chapter 6

POPULATIONS AT RISK

Exposure in different agricultural systems

For several reasons, the use of pesticides and thus the possible health effects, differ between regions and farming systems. In developing countries most of the farmers cater for local needs only. There may be many pest problems in this type of agriculture, but usually the losses are "accepted" or controlled in traditional ways. Use of pesticides is limited, as the farmers are either not aware of their existence, or cannot afford them, or do not feel that they are of value.

In developing countries with commercial agriculture, some pesticides may find their way into the hands of the subsistence farmers, who are unfamiliar with the potential risks and necessary safety measures.

The use of pesticides in agriculture in developing countries is thus very much connected with production for the regional, national, or international markets. As shown in Table 7 (page 28), the most intensive use of pesticides is in the production of horticultural crops, cotton, soya beans, rice, corn and wheat.

Farming systems in developing countries can be categorized in many ways, according to crops, water conditions, method of cultivation, nutrient supply, and degree of commercialization. For this discussion, the three categories defined by Copplestone (1985) will be used. These are: plantation farming, which tends to be monocultural and requires intensive pest control; cash-cropping, which is diverse in both the types of crop grown and the size of the holdings; and subsistence farming. Migratory workers often play an important role in these systems. The smaller the holding and the more the crop is for subsistence, the lower is the likelihood that pesticides will be used. The crop itself also has an influence, the two crops most vulnerable to insect attack being cotton and rice. Herbicides tend to be less widely used in all types of agriculture in developing areas, since weeds can be controlled by human effort, although Papua New Guinea is a notable exception (Mowbray, 1988).

In plantations, employees may be provided with housing, food, and some medical care. Plantations vary in the care and training provided and sometimes set their own standards rather than conform to any minimum national standard of working conditions. Pesticide use may be high but the amount of exposure usually depends on the quality of management. Pesticides are often used on a large scale using aircraft or tractor-driven equipment.

On most farms with cash-crops the situation is different in many respects. Many cash-crop farms are family affairs, while on others families, rather than individuals, are employed to carry out the routine operations. Thus, large sections of the rural population are involved. In some developing countries, these people may make up more than half the total rural population, excluding plantation workers and those too old or too young to work in the fields or look after the flocks. In general, the cash-cropping farmers use smaller quantities of pesticides than the plantation farmers, either because of lack of access or because of the high cost.

As pointed out by Copplestone (1985), the likelihood of exposure to pesticides depends on family structure and traditional living habits. Where the farmers and their families live close to the fields the risk of exposure is higher than where they live in villages and walk long distances to their work.

For subsistence farmers, there is much less exposure to pesticides because usually they cannot afford the products. They must suffer the crop losses caused by pests, and probably represent the group least exposed to pesticides (Copplestone, 1985).

The most important crops with respect to pesticide use are cotton, rice, and maize. Certain plantation crops such as fruits, coffee, and tea are also important, but they are grown on much smaller areas. In the developing parts of the world, cotton, rice, and maize are grown on 27, 140, and 80 million hectares, respectively. Coffee plantations make up another 10.5 million hectares. More details are shown in Table 24.

However, only a small part of the rice and maize production can be regarded as pesticide-intensive. Most of these crops are

Table 24. Total area of agricultural land and areas occupied by certain crops, by economic class and region, 1985 (million hectares)[a]

Class and region	Agricultural land	Cotton	Rice paddy	Maize	Coffee
Developed market economies	399	4.8	3.8	43	–
Developing market economies	684	21.3	102	62	10.4
Africa	153	3.1	5.0	16	3.7
Latin America	177	5.3	7.0	28	5.7
Eastern Mediterranean	82	1.9	1.1	2.2	–
East Asia	271	11.0	86.6	16	1.0
Others	1	–	2.4	–	0.04
Centrally planned economies	391	9.1	41	28	0.04
Asia	114	5.8	40	18	0.04
Eastern Europe and USSR	277	3.3	0.7	10	–
All developed countries	676	8.1	4.5	53	–
All developing countries	798	27.1	142	80	10.5

[a] Source: FAO, 1986b.

grown by subsistence farmers, who produce most of the food in the developing world.

In many developing countries, pesticide use is rapidly becoming more common, even in production for the local markets. Production is becoming more intensive, and fertilizers, pesticides, and new varieties of crops are widely used. These developments are often supported by national agricultural extension programmes and the number of people exposed to pesticides is steadily increasing.

About 20% of all pesticides are sold in developing countries. Most of the active ingredients are manufactured in developed countries and are shipped either in this form for local formulation, or as formulated concentrates. Insecticides, fungicides, and rodenticides make up a higher proportion of the total in developing countries, since these are used for the control of the major pests in these areas.

On plantations the proportion of the staff exposed to highly concentrated materials for relatively long periods throughout the growing season tends to be low (perhaps 10–25%), because the staff have more specialized functions. Most of the people engaged in cash-cropping, especially those working on small farms, may use pesticides at least for part of the growing season. In plantations and cash-cropping farms, most of those engaged in field work and harvesting will have some contact with pesticide residues, but the exposure of workers engaged in crop production to pesticides that quickly degrade can be reduced by appropriate "waiting times" after each pesticide application.

Exposure in public health programmes

Of the pesticides destined for non-agricultural purposes, many are used by governments in public health programmes, frequently for the control of vector-borne diseases. The insecticides used are mainly for the control of malaria, filariasis, and trypanosomiasis; molluscicides are also used fairly widely in some places for schistosomiasis control (Copplestone, 1985). Rodenticides not only protect food stores but also contribute to the prevention of plague. The use of pesticides in public health gives rise to the possibility of exposure of the spraying staff and of the general public.

In general, a limited range of pesticides is used and their toxicity is also limited; the inevitable exposure of the general public in the spraying of households in villages and the use of space sprays and fogs in urban areas limit the choice of pesticide and formulation. However, the spray operators may continue applying pesticides for weeks or months, on an almost daily basis.

Although staff may be involved in spraying for long periods, they are usually employed on a daily basis; their wages are low and they are likely to have received little education. They are given basic training in spraying techniques, but training in safety practices is often neglected so as not to alarm them unduly. Frequently, they receive neither guidance nor a good example from their supervisors. However, they are usually exposed only to compounds of low toxicity, as recommended for public health use (Copplestone, 1985).

Size of populations at risk

In developing countries, the proportion of the population dependent on agriculture is generally high (Table 25). On average, 63% of the economically active members of the population work in the agricultural sector. The corresponding figure for developed countries is 11%. Thus, even if pesticide use in developing areas is low, relatively more people are involved in the handling of pesticides, or live in areas where pesticides are used in agriculture.

Table 25. Total population, agricultural population, and economically active population by economic class and region, 1985 (in millions)[a]

Class and region	Total population	Agricultural population	Economically active population		
			Total	In agriculture	Percentage in agriculture
Developed market economies	818	57	378	25	6.7
North America	264	8.5	130	4.2	3.2
Western Europe	378	33	167	14	8.6
Australia and New Zealand	19	1.4	8.8	0.6	7.1
Israel, Japan and South Africa	157	14	72	6.2	8.6
Developing market economies	2478	1387	923	528	57
Africa	451	307	182	128	71
Latin America	405	115	140	39	28
Eastern Mediterranean	242	102	77	33	44
East Asia	1375	860	522	326	63
Others	5.8	3.2	2.4	1.4	58
Centrally planned economies	1541	885	862	505	59
Asia	1149	814	660	469	71
Eastern Europe and USSR	392	71	202	36	18
All developed countries	1210	128	580	62	11
All developing countries	3627	2201	1583	998	63

[a] Source: FAO, 1986b.

The United Republic of Tanzania, for example, has a population of 22 million, and 90% of the people live in the rural areas. The economically active population is about 10 million, of which 8 million make up the rural workforce. The different categories of agricultural workers are distributed as follows: plantation workers and wage earners, 1.5%; mixed farming, rearing livestock, hunting, and fishing, 6%; and subsistence farming and cash-crop production, 92% (J. Nkurlu, personal communication, 1987).

In some developing countries, estimations have been made of the exposure to pesticides of different groups in the rural population. For instance, in Sichuan Province in China, with a population of about 87 million, the total area of the agricultural land is 6.5 million hectares. The amount of pesticide used on average is 4 kg per hectare. About 10 million people (12% of the population) are involved in the use of pesticides each year. From a survey of 78 000 people (F. Xu, personal communication, 1987), it was estimated that in the whole province, the number of people affected by poisoning each year would be 100 000 among the 10 million using pesticides (1%). The pesticides that caused most poisoning were the organophosphorus compounds (77%), and the main route of exposure was dermal (60–65%).

These data indicate that about 5–10% of the agricultural population in certain developing countries are likely to have significant exposure to pesticides. This figure may also be calculated from the total area of land used for agriculture that depends on pesticides. Cotton production occupies 27 million hectares in the developing world (Table 24) and production is pesticide-intensive. Coffee plantations, another pesticide-intensive crop, occupy about 10 million hectares. Other pesticide-intensive crops include tea, vegetables, and fruits, which together cover a few million hectares. The intensive use of pesticides in rice and maize production is limited to a small part of the total production in the developing countries. These figures mean that the agricultural land under intensive pesti-cide use in the developing countries totals about 40 million hectares, or about 5% of the agricultural land, including the plantation areas. This implies that about 50 million of the economically active population, or about 100 million of the "agricultural population" (5% of 2200 million, Table 25), are likely to be involved in agriculture with intensive pesticide use or be living in areas where such agriculture takes place.

In addition, as much as 50% of the rural economically active population may be involved in cash-cropping in some coun-tries. Thus, 500 million people may be exposed to pesticides to a lesser extent.

As pointed out earlier, the situation in many developing countries is changing rapidly. New types of agricultural production lead to more pesticide use. The population figures estimated here are thus also likely to increase.

The non-agricultural population in developing countries (1400 million people) will be exposed to pesticides mainly as residues in food and occasionally as the result of disease vector control operations.

Chapter 7

PUBLIC HEALTH IMPACT

The preceding chapters have shown that acute poisoning—including suicide attempts, mass poisonings from contaminated food, chemical accidents in industry, and occupational exposure in agriculture—is the cause of most of the serious health effects associated with pesticides. Chronic effects, including cancer, adverse reproductive outcome, and immunological effects, are also of potential public health concern, in view of the large body of experimental animal data and the few epidemiological studies so far carried out.

Acute effects in individuals

Hard data from which the annual incidence of cases of acute, fatal and non-fatal pesticide poisoning could be estimated are not available. However, models and informal estimates based on hospitalization data and population surveys (WHO, 1986a) suggest that the annual incidence of cases of unintentional acute poisoning with severe manifestations probably exceeds 1 million (1985), with a case-fatality rate of 0.4–1.9% (Table 26). Other published estimates range from 750 000 (Bull, 1982) to 2 000 000 cases (ESCAP, 1983). Occupational exposure is estimated to account for 70% (700 000 cases) of the cases of severe unintentional poisoning. It has been estimated that there are an additional 2 million cases of intentional poisoning (mainly suicide attempts) (Jeyaratnam, 1985). Of the more than 220 000 intentional and unintentional deaths from acute poisoning, suicides account for approximately 91%, occupational exposure for 6%, and other causes, including food contamination, for 3% (Jeyaratnam, 1985).

The WHO estimate of an annual total of 1 million cases of unintentional poisoning includes hospitalized and non-hospitalized cases, the number of the latter being calculated on the basis of 6 non-hospitalized (unreported) cases to each hospitalized (reported) case. Other proportions ranging from 10:1 (Jeyaratnam et al., 1987) to 100:1 (Kahn, 1976) have been suggested from surveys of pesticide poisoning. The

Table 26. Published global estimates of the annual number of cases of pesticide poisoning

Year	Cases	Deaths	Reference
Unintentional poisonings			
1973	500 000	–	WHO, 1973
1977	–	20 640	Copplestone, 1977
1985	1 111 000	20 000	Levine, 1986 (area surveys of mortality: method used in the study by WHO, 1973)
1985	1 000 000	20 000	WHO, 1986a
Intentional poisonings (suicides)			
1985	2 000 000	200 000	Jeyaratnam (1985) (based on hospital data)

number of less severe poisonings may therefore be much greater than that estimated by WHO. The case–fatality rate is another way of estimating the occurrence of poisoning. In the WHO report, it was estimated as 1 in 50 (hospitalized and non-hospitalized cases), whereas in a study of isomalathion poisoning in Pakistan (Baker et al., 1978) the case-fatality rate for symptomatic cases (questionnaire study) was 1 in 500. Estimates of the total number of cases of pesticide poisoning, including all severity levels, based on the greatest of these multipliers, suggest that the number of cases may be much greater than the approximately 3 million severe cases specified in Table 26.

Another method of calculating the number of cases of pesticide poisoning is based on the size of the population at risk as estimated in Chapter 6. According to Jeyaratnam et al. (1987), in some countries about 7% of workers involved in agriculture with intensive pesticide use may experience symptoms of poisoning each year (including cases of mild poisoning), if effective training programmes are not in place. This estimate does not include suicide attempts. One estimate from China suggested that 1% of all pesticide users in agriculture could be poisoned each year. The size of the population in developing countries with intensive exposure was estimated at 50 million and a total of 500 million people may have a lower level of exposure to pesticides. This would mean that there could be 3.5–5 million cases of unintentional poisonings each year (including both mild and severe poisoning), but all such estimates are uncertain.

Mass poisonings

The recorded outbreaks of mass poisoning caused by contaminated food have resulted in about 15 000 cases in 41 years or 366 cases per year, a relatively small contribution to the total number of cases of acute poisoning. The extent of under-reporting is not known, but it is likely that large-scale epidemic outbreaks do become known.

Chronic effects

Lack of data precludes any estimation of the number of people with chronic health effects. Pesticides have been implicated in various disorders and diseases, including cancer, adverse reproductive outcomes, peripheral neuropathies, neurobehavioural disorders, impaired immune function, and allergic sensitization reactions, particularly of the skin. Cumulative inhibition of cholinesterase activity as a result of long-term, low-dose exposure to organophosphorus compounds lowers the threshold for acute poisoning from such insecticides. Dehydration and poor nutrition also appear to lower the toxicity threshold to these pesticides.

The possibility of chronic health effects following pesticide exposure is supported by a large body of data from laboratory animals. However, as pointed out in Chapter 4, epidemiological data are available for only some of the effects. The documented effects include male sterility from exposure to DBCP and neurobehavioural disorders from low-level, long-term exposure to organophosphorus compounds. Peripheral neuropathies have been observed for a small number of pesticides. Proliferative lung disease has been known to result from exposure to paraquat (dermal exposure or ingestion). Allergic sensitization dermatoses have been related to a number of pesticides, and persistent neuropsychiatric effects following acute pesticide poisoning have been observed in a small percentage of cases.

For primary contact dermatitis and neurobehavioural impairment following acute poisoning, the limited data permit some preliminary estimates of the likelihood of chronic health effects after exposure to pesticides, in groups with occupational exposure in agriculture. On the basis of experience in California, USA (CDFA, 1986), where it was found that the number of dermatoses caused by pesticides among agricultural workers was the same as the number of severe unintentional occupational poisonings, it can be estimated that 700 000 cases may occur annually throughout the world (see page 85). If it is assumed that 70% of acute occupational poisonings are caused by organophosphorus compounds (Jeyaratnam et al., 1987) and that 5% of these poisonings will lead to persistent neuro-behavioural effects (Eskenazi & Maizlish, 1988), there would be 25 000 such cases each year. Using the same assumptions for other unintentional poisonings, an annual figure of 10 000 can be calculated on the basis of the 300 000 severe cases (page 85).

In some occupational groups exposed to certain pesticides, e.g. farmers or pesticide manufacturers, epidemiological studies have demonstrated an increased risk of lung cancer, lympho-poietic cancers, and possibly other forms of cancer. In addition, there is a potential cancer risk from ingesting certain pesticides.

A calculation based on a linear-risk extrapolation from animal data and exposure at the maximum tolerated USA residue levels for 28 pesticides (NAS, 1987), for the 550 million people with high or intermediate exposure, indicates the possibility of about 37 000 cases of cancer each year in developing countries. Considering the size of the population with potential exposure, the calculated number of cases is relatively small, particularly when compared with the number of acute poisonings. It should be noted that in developing countries certain pesticides (e.g., organochlorine compounds) are used that are not used in the USA. This factor would probably add substantially to the estimate. However, many of the pesticides presumed to be carcinogenic that were included in the calculation model used by NAS are not genotoxic and, for them, the mechanism of carcinogenicity is unclear.

In the absence of data, it is not possible to estimate the number of cases of adverse reproductive outcome, peripheral neuropathy, impaired immune function, including skin sensitization, and neurobehavioural effects associated with low-level, long-term pesticide exposure.

Assessment of overall public health impact

No segment of the general population is completely protected against exposure to pesticides and potentially serious health effects, although a disproportionate burden is shouldered by the people of the developing world and by high-risk groups in each country.

Fig. 6. Estimated overall annual public health impact of pesticide poisoning

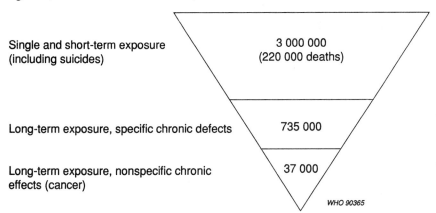

Single and short-term exposure (including suicides)

3 000 000 (220 000 deaths)

Long-term exposure, specific chronic defects

735 000

Long-term exposure, nonspecific chronic effects (cancer)

37 000

WHO 90365

The estimated 3 million cases of severe acute poisoning (Fig. 6) may be matched by a greater number of unreported, but mild cases of intoxication and acute conditions such as dermatitis. The estimates in Fig. 6 of the number of cases of chronic effects are smaller than the number of acute effects, which inverts the pyramid in Fig. 2 (page 13). The high levels of acute and chronic morbidity emphasize the need for medical and rehabilitation services. An unknown number of less serious health effects may add to the overall disease burden, but precise estimates must await future epidemiological studies.

Future trends in public health impact

If, as expected, the use of chemical pesticides doubles in the next ten years in developing countries and if agricultural practices continue to develop, it is likely that the number of cases of intentional and unintentional acute poisoning will increase accordingly, unless major educational and preventive programmes are introduced. The greatest increase in pesticide use is expected to be in the use of herbicides. Organochlorine pesticides will be less used but insecticidal organophosphorus compounds and insecticidal/nematocidal carbamates are increasing in importance. Unless the use of the most toxic pesticides is reduced, the risks of acute intoxication will increase. With the increased emphasis on cash-crops and plantation-style farming in developing countries, the number of individuals in high-risk occupations may increase over the next decade despite a decrease in the proportion of the overall population directly involved in agricultural production.

Chapter 8

APPROACHES TO THE PREVENTION OF PESTICIDE POISONING

The estimates in Chapter 7 show clearly that a major effort is required to prevent the millions of cases of pesticide poisoning that occur every year. The problem of suicide attempts is perhaps most serious; one contribution to prevention would involve making highly toxic pesticides less easily available to people not actually engaged in their application. For the reduction of unintentional poisonings, a number of different approaches are needed. The dearth of epidemiological data has hitherto contributed to the lack of assertive and effective action to prevent pesticide poisoning. However, such action can and should be taken on the basis of the available toxicological knowledge. For example, the choice of less toxic pesticides and the use of standard protective procedures during pesticide application would prevent much pesticide poisoning.

Particular problems of pesticide safety in developing countries

Hazards arising during the application of pesticides are mainly due to lack of information, knowledge, and awareness, poor supervision during spraying, absence of proper legislation or of enforcement of legislation, and sale on the open market of highly toxic pesticides. Compliance with the available guidelines for the safe use of pesticides (e.g., ILO, 1977; WHO, 1985; FAO, 1985a) would control most of these hazards.

The manufacturer, formulator, or person responsible for labelling and registering a pesticide with the appropriate national authority, should ensure that the product offered for sale, or otherwise distributed, bears a label written in the language of the region, giving comprehensive instructions for safe use, warning of possible hazards, specifying the active ingredients, as well as all other ingredients, and giving guidelines for first aid in case of poisoning (including antidotes).

Although considerable amounts of pesticide are imported from industrialized countries, it is to be expected that more developing countries will in the future manufacture their own pesticides and prepare their own formulations. It will then be the responsibility of the governments to enforce good manufacturing practice and quality control, and to ensure proper use of the product. To meet this responsibility, the authorities must set up chemical, analytical, and toxicological facilities, and be able to monitor exposure to pesticides.

Collaboration could be established with developed countries, but eventually it will be essential for countries to achieve self-sufficiency. Coordination will be needed between the government departments dealing with health, agriculture, the environment, and occupational hygiene, so that all aspects related to pesticides used in public health and agriculture can be covered nationally in a single set of requirements (WHO, 1982a).

The Food and Agriculture Organization of the United Nations (FAO), in consultation with appropriate United Nations agencies and other organizations, has prepared a Code of Conduct on the Distribution and Use of Pesticides, based on internationally agreed technical guidelines. This Code was adopted by the Twenty-third Session of the FAO Conference in November 1985 (FAO, 1986a). It defines the responsibilities of, and establishes voluntary standards of conduct for, the various sectors of society (including government and industry), in order to reduce the hazards associated with the introduction, distribution, and use of pesticides. The Code also defines the conditions under which different pesticides may be used efficiently while minimizing risks to human health and the environment. One of the basic functions of the Code, which is voluntary, is to serve as a point of reference, particularly until countries have established adequate regulatory infrastructures for pesticide management.

The World Bank has recommended that projects involving pesticides of the highest hazard level (class Ia and Ib) should not be supported unless suitable precautions are guaranteed (World Bank, 1985).

Improving pesticide use, and alternative strategies for pest control

Good agricultural practice (GAP) in the use of pesticides is defined by FAO as "the officially recommended or authorized usage of a pesticide under practical conditions at any stage of production, storage, transport, distribution and processing of food and other agricultural commodities, bearing in mind the variations in requirements within and between regions, and which takes into account the minimum quantities necessary to achieve adequate control, the pesticide being applied in a manner so as to leave a residue which is the smallest amount practicable and which is toxicologically acceptable" (FAO, 1977).

Pest management may comprise many different methods varying from routine applications of pesticides to subtle measures for ecological management. The concept of pest control based solely on the use of pesticides is being abandoned in most countries. It is increasingly being recognized that maximum use should be made of naturally occurring, or introduced, biological agents that can help to limit the abundance of pest organisms and the incidence of plant or animal diseases. This concept is an element of Integrated Pest Control (FAO, 1967) or Integrated Pest Management (IPM) defined as "a pest management system that, in the context of the associated environment and the population dynamics of the pest species, utilizes all suitable techniques and methods in as compatible a manner as possible and maintains the pest population at levels below those causing economic injury" (Balk & Koeman, 1984). IPM has been tested systematically in a number of countries and has provided the most effective and economical control (FAO, 1979).

Much has been learnt about minimizing environmental pollution by pesticides since the period after the Second World War, when many persistent pesticides were used in a relatively haphazard and indiscriminate way. At that time, aerial spraying of large areas of land was common. Now, in the developed countries, such aerial spraying is subject to considerable constraints and legislation. However, it is still used to some extent in developing countries, often because of the poorer communication systems.

Whenever possible, biological control measures should be used, although the extent to which these can provide the necessary pest control may be limited. However, there have been a number of successes, particularly in relation to pests introduced from other countries. Pheromones are becoming increasingly useful, especially for lepidopterous pests, and considerable progress has been made with control of cutworms. One of the main problems with pheromones is their high degree of specificity and the need for a different pheromone for every pest. The release of sterile males is very effective for certain pests, such as the tsetse fly.

Although biological control methods are sometimes not adequate to control major pests, they can be incorporated into integrated control and pest management schemes to provide very satisfactory control with minimal environmental problems. Growers in developing countries seem to be very receptive to community and other non-chemical control techniques. More-over, where these methods are labour-intensive, this is not such a problem as it would be in developed countries. There is great scope for the development of improved pest management in developing countries and there should be greatly increased promotion of such projects (Edwards, 1977b).

Legislation

In the developed countries, stringent legal requirements regarding toxicological and ecological effects have to be satisfied before the importation and use of any particular pesticide is permitted. The costs of satisfying these requirements, when a new pesticide is being developed, are very high, running into millions of dollars. This is reflected by the fact that few new compounds reach the market annually, because the high cost of development requires a large and certain market for any new pesticide.

Before approving the use of a specific pesticide, the responsible government agency may require that the manufacturer provides data from standard animal toxicity tests and from field studies of ecological effects and environmental transfer.

Although the results of animal tests provide a reasonably good indication of the potential hazard of a chemical to human health, there is still a need to survey human populations for evidence of any ill-effects of chemical exposure. This is because different species may have different responses to a particular chemical, and also because an infrequent effect that becomes apparent only in a large population could well be missed in tests on a limited number of animals. These two difficulties are generally expected to be overcome by the use of an adequate safety factor in setting exposure limits. It is important to realize, however, that epidemiological studies can only be carried out after the product has been released on to the market, because human exposure before then is extremely limited. Most epidemiological studies have been carried out in occupational situations, where a well defined human population has a clearly defined exposure.

The fact that a developing country may have a real need for hazardous compounds in no way detracts from its responsibility to see that these are used safely, and do not result in cases of accidental poisoning, especially when they are used occupationally. Possibly the most effective single measure would be to restrict the use of the most hazardous compounds to teams, governmental or private, who have been specially trained in application and whose work practices and precautions can be regularly checked. Such a restriction could, for example, be applied to all formulations in Class Ia and Class Ib of the WHO Recommended Classification of Pesticides by Hazard (Table 16). This does not mean that the restriction should apply to all technical products listed in Class Ia and Class Ib of the Classification. All classification must be by formulation, and formulations of technical products with a low concentration of active ingredient may well fall into a lower hazard class. Plestina (1984) proposed that availability of insecticides be restricted according to hazard class (Table 27).

Education, training, and information

Misuse of pesticides is often the result of ignorance, which can only be dealt with by education and training. There are many ways to approach this: through education and training of health and agricultural workers who have leadership roles in their community, through radio broadcasts, through farmers'

Table 27. Recommended restrictions on availability of insecticides[a]

Class		Available to:
Ia	Extremely hazardous	Individually licensed operators only
Ib	Highly hazardous	Well trained, educated, strictly supervised operators
II	Moderately hazardous	Trained and supervised operators who are known to observe strict precautionary measures
III	Slightly hazardous	Trained operators who observe routine precautionary measures
–	Unlikely to present acute hazard in normal use	General public respecting standard general hygienic measures and observing instructions for use given on the label

[a] Source: Plestina, 1984

groups or cooperatives, through retailers, or through other community leaders. Training courses for trainers can make use of WHO multilevel training modules (WHO, 1978b, 1980) and other suitable texts (Plestina, 1984). Training materials are also available from UNEP, FAO, the International Group of National Associations of Manufacturers of Agrochemical Products (GIFAP, Brussels, Belgium) and the International Organization of Consumers Unions (IOCU, The Hague, Netherlands).

The most practical and simple way of imparting information, at present, is the label. However, the label required by many registration authorities now contains so much detail that it is often self-defeating (GIFAP, 1988). A separate simple pictorial safety label would therefore be most useful (Fig. 7). This should clearly indicate by colour the hazard class, and by symbol, the precautions to be taken (Copplestone, 1985).

The skull and crossbones symbol should be reserved for formulations in classes Ia and Ib, with the words "Very toxic" and "Toxic", as appropriate. The cross should be used for hazard class II with the word "Harmful". Class III is denoted by the word "Caution". This simple symbol and wording system has been recommended by FAO and WHO.

It is important to remember that a large proportion of those who make day-to-day decisions on agricultural operations will have had little education and may be unable to read. It is sometimes overlooked that inability to read in rural populations in many parts of the world is accompanied by difficulty in interpreting pictures. The people may not have been exposed to television, for instance, which in many developing

Fig. 7. Warning symbols and text recommended by FAO for use on pesticide packaging[a]

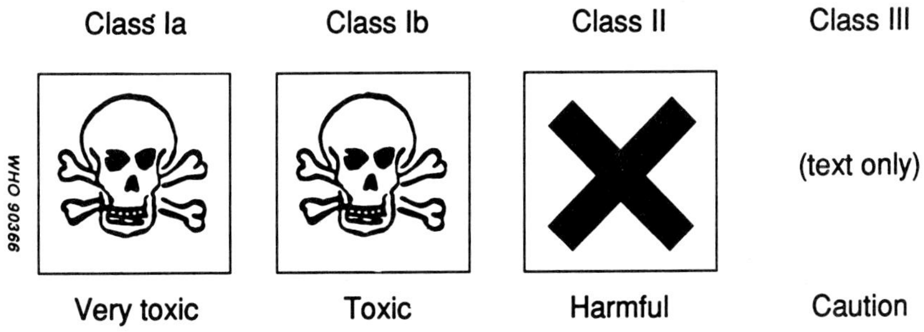

Class Ia	Class Ib	Class II	Class III

Very toxic	Toxic	Harmful	Caution

[a] From FAO (1985b)

countries is found only in the cities. Formal education may have been limited to religious subjects, and have involved learning by rote, without pictorial representations to assist. Communication may take place only through the spoken word, but this does not necessarily depend on personal contact, as the radio and the telephone are generally understood and used. In these situations, extension services can play an important role in bringing information and education to the users of pesticides (Edwards, 1977b).

In the absence of a national infrastructure for pesticide control activities, responsibility for education may rest with the vendor of the pesticide (Copplestone, 1985). It is important that personnel all the way down the distribution chain should be aware of the hazards, as well as the uses, of the products they are selling. They should pass on advice appropriate to the hazard, and should not pretend that hazardous pesticides can be used without precautions. The more toxic the pesticide, the greater is the user's need for adequate advice and the responsibility of the vendor to give it.

Agricultural medicine

The establishment of a suitable infrastructure to ensure that the adverse effects of pesticides on both the human population and the environment are minimized will need efforts in all areas of pest management and pesticide control. In addition, emphasis should be placed on the occupational health of workers in the agricultural sector, with appropriate medical surveillance and record-keeping (WHO, 1982a). The following points should be considered:

● Greater emphasis should be placed on the occupational health of workers in the agricultural sector in both developing and developed countries.

● In developing countries, the training of general practitioners should stress the need to integrate occupational health with public health programmes, especially primary health care.

● The scope of health problems in the agricultural sector should be defined through appropriate surveys to determine (*a*) the types and amounts of pesticide used, (*b*) the current state of health of workers in relation to pesticide exposure, and (*c*) the number, sex, and age of the workers exposed.

● A system of priorities should be established, to ensure that available resources are used to solve the most pressing and critical problems.

Coordination between hospital physicians, occupational health specialists, and primary health care staff is needed to standardize the way in which information about workers hospitalized or treated for pesticide exposure is monitored and reported. Data obtained from clinical examinations should be used to develop occupational health limits. Comprehensive occupational health histories should be obtained from all workers adversely affected by pesticide exposure (WHO, 1982a).

Research needs

Development of less hazardous pesticides

Pesticides can be made less hazardous by the use of less toxic active ingredients and solvents, and formulations that are more dilute and that are not readily absorbed through the skin or by inhalation.

Experimental data

In the absence of data from human studies, or where information on human effects is limited, long-term animal studies are needed. Studies using both male and female experimental animals are essential to permit assessment of the effects of pesticide exposure on reproductive function. Guidelines should be developed for the evaluation and extrapolation of animal data and internationally acceptable criteria should be established for the selection of animal models and extrapolation procedures (WHO, 1982a). There is also a need for the increased use of *in vitro* studies to elucidate the mechanisms of action of various pesticides. In a critical appraisal of short-term assays for carcinogenicity (IARC, 1980), it was concluded that, intelligently used, such assays have several advantages. They may be of importance for the planning of long-term animal assays and for evaluation of the results. They may contribute to better design of epidemiological studies, and can be useful in ascertaining the absence of certain adverse effects in the development of new pesticides.

Metabolic studies

Additional studies are needed to increase the validity of the methods used for biological monitoring and to obtain further data on the metabolism of pesticides. Studies of percutaneous absorption, taking into account the vehicle, the site of exposure, and the sex and age of the person, are needed to identify metabolites suitable for use in the screening of exposed workers (WHO, 1982a).

Residue monitoring programmes

In North America and Europe, pesticide residues in the physical environment and in plants and animals are closely monitored. In developing countries, such surveys are only just beginning and there is a need for more data on the levels and persistence of pesticide residues in the tropics.

To prevent any harmful effects on the environment, the levels of pesticide residues in air, soil, and water should be monitored regularly. The monitoring of pesticide residues in food is one of the most important approaches to minimizing the potential hazards to human health. When unacceptable levels of pesticides are found, appropriate steps should be taken to identify the cause and to prevent recurrence.

People in developing countries tend to have a larger body burden of pesticides than do people in developed countries. Regular monitoring of residues in human tissues, followed when necessary by appropriate preventive action, would be useful.

Epidemiological studies

Epidemiological studies are severely hampered by the lack of valid data on people exposed to pesticides under field conditions or during manufacture or formulation. Emphasis should be placed on the design of studies meeting well defined principles and design criteria; such studies should include, as a minimum, (a) environmental monitoring, (b) biological monitoring, and (c) evaluation of health effects. Data on health effects obtained in the clinical setting should be well documented and supported with detailed exposure histories. These proposals were originally made in the context of occupational exposures (WHO, 1982a), but they are equally valid for exposures in other situations. In addition, the concepts and terminology used should conform with modern principles developed internationally (Last, 1988).

Effective research on long-term health hazards of exposure to pesticides will necessitate changes in the direction and emphasis of epidemiological research, particularly as regards cancer, reproductive effects, and neurobehavioural effects (Sharp et al., 1986). The present epidemiological approach to detecting pesticides that represent a hazard as regards human cancer is hampered by two major factors. First, many human cancers cannot be detected for 20 years or more after exposure. This problem has led to increasing reliance being placed on animal studies. However, the use of genetically pure strains of animals in constant environmental conditions and on controlled diets may not detect the hazard for human subjects, particularly if the interaction of several agents and conditions is involved. Secondly, exposure to particular chemicals, at least in industrialized countries, is declining with improved industrial practices and increasing environmental awareness. While this trend is highly desirable, it reduces the likelihood of an effect being detected in epidemiological studies. Therefore, it is imperative to investigate biological markers of early change that can be tested in exposed populations.

In the past, many studies of reproductive hazards concentrated on groups of the general population with low exposure to the pesticide in question. Such studies will continue to give controversial results because of the multiple comparisons involved and the uncertainty regarding exposure levels. Emphasis should be placed on high-exposure groups (particularly occupational groups) and on the development of valid methods for extrapolation to groups with low exposure.

Surveillance of potential high-risk groups is needed, and is easy to implement with regard to congenital defects and stillbirth rates. More sensitive indices, such as early spontaneous abortion and sperm deficiencies, may be necessary in specific circumstances, but the cost and personal resistance to participation generally render such techniques impracticable on a large scale.

DBCP (1,2-dibromo-3-chloropropane) is the only pesticide that has been shown to have a clear effect on reproduction in human beings. This may be simply because occupational studies have concentrated on men. The greater participation of women in the workforce should result in more epidemiological studies being carried out on women exposed to pesticides. Future epidemiological studies on the reproductive hazards of pesticides should concentrate on identifying exposed women, particularly in agricultural work.

Epidemiological research on neurotoxic effects will be necessary to clarify the relationship between pesticides and neuro-behavioural deficits, particularly when routine neurological testing or biological monitoring fails to detect abnormalities during chronic low-level exposure. Such research may well have important implications for medical surveillance and worker protection (Sharp et al., 1986).

Chapter 9

PROPOSALS FOR FUTURE EPIDEMIOLOGICAL RESEARCH

Few data are available on the occurrence of pesticide-related illness among defined populations, particularly in the developing world. Baseline descriptive epidemiological data on the extent of pesticide poisoning in developing countries are urgently needed.

In addition, there is a need for increased national awareness of control requirements for diseases associated with pesticide exposure, and for the development of specific mechanisms to achieve national multisectoral collaboration and good communication with international agencies. Basic national exposure-assessment data (i.e., types and amounts of pesticides produced, imported, or formulated in the country, and places of sale) should be compiled in each country.

Development of "area profiles" and descriptive data relating to acute poisoning

It may be necessary, as part of such projects, to conduct a census of the population being surveyed in order to ensure that adequate descriptive data are available for the detailed epidemiological analysis.

Within each defined population, an "area profile" should then be developed, containing the following information:

- Descriptive demographic characteristics of the community (age, sex, race, ethnicity, marital status, education, occupation, religion, and income).

- Descriptive information on the leading causes of mortality and morbidity within the community.

- Agricultural and geographical characteristics (types of crops produced, extent to which crops are consumed locally or exported, destinations of exported crops, characteristics of climate and terrain that may affect pesticide toxicity and/or exposure).

- Data on pesticides used (types and quantities used for each crop, projections for the future based on past and current data).

- Environmental pesticide levels and human exposure (air, soil, water, crop levels in the fields, residues in food, effects of such factors as rainfall and temperature).

- Activities and practices leading to occupational exposure (formulation, mixing, loading, applying, farming, food handling).

- Sources of non-occupational exposure (restrictions on pesticide availability, labelling, storage, transport, disposal and sales practices, potential use for suicide attempts).

- Biological monitoring of exposure (specific quantitative assessments—e.g., circulating cholinesterase and/or pesticide levels, urinary metabolites, pesticide levels in human milk and in adipose tissue).

- Data on morbidity and mortality (including suicides) due to acute pesticide poisoning, covering a period sufficient to allow for the assessment of all seasonal cycles within the community (formulation of specific case-definitions and diagnostic criteria; development of a surveillance network for the complete coverage of records from all hospitals, poison centres and outpatient centres serving the defined population; development of quality control and data handling procedures that will ensure the timely availability of surveillance information).

- Characteristics of poisoning cases (demographic profile, medical history, crop exposure, pesticides used, personal degree of environmental exposure, source of pesticide causing the poisoning episode, and mechanism of exposure). This information should be used to facilitate detection of new cases and initiation of appropriate preventive interventions.

- Number and geographical location of facilities for the treatment of pesticide illness (emergency rooms, clinics, etc.) and the number of health workers trained in the recognition, treatment, and control of pesticide poisoning.

Evaluation of interventions for acute poisoning

Once an area profile has been completed, sufficient information should be available for the development of intervention strategies designed to lower the incidence of acute pesticide poisoning in the target community. Such strategies should be formulated so as to permit testing of hypotheses regarding knowledge, attitudes, behaviour and/or other determinants of pesticide exposure (e.g., wearing of protective clothing or legislative approaches). Moreover, the area profile should be maintained and updated, in order to determine whether the primary objective—reduction of the incidence of acute pesticide poisoning—is being met.

Once the intervention strategy has been shown to be successful, the project should be expanded to other high-risk areas within the country.

Studies of chronic effects

While acute pesticide poisoning produces a dramatic and often catastrophic immediate outcome, the chronic effects that may result from long-term exposure are also of concern throughout the world.

The methods required to study the chronic effects are somewhat different from those used in studies of acute effects. First, it is necessary to develop a method for long-term individual follow-up. In some situations, when the effects are easily diagnosed in a standardized way, case–control studies may be used, but this would require the availability of well-defined control groups. Secondly, the present and past exposure levels must be quantified. New approaches to biological monitoring, using the markers mentioned earlier, will be required. Without valid measurements of exposure covering relatively long periods, studies of chronic effects cannot be carried out. Modern pesticides that are rapidly detoxified in the environment, and for which there is no evidence of chronic effects from animal studies, may be of low priority for studies of chronic effects when resources are limited.

In view of the lack of epidemiological data, it is clearly in the interest of both the public health community and the pesticide industry to invest in more epidemiological studies of well-defined, exposed groups. Studies in which sensitive tests do not find any effects will help to reassure the users of pesticides. Studies that do find effects will, on the other hand, help in the design of immediate preventive measures, and the setting of safety standards for the future.

Chapter 10

RECOMMENDATIONS

Control of acute pesticide poisoning

Efforts are needed on the part of national authorities, non-governmental organizations and industry to control the major problem of acute pesticide poisoning, particularly in the developing countries. To this end the following steps should be taken.

- Training and information activities on pesticide safety should be established and strengthened.

- Legislation to control the use of pesticides and to set up the infrastructure for enforcement should be established and harmonized.

- Systems need to be developed for obtaining descriptive epidemiological data on acute pesticide poisoning to be used as baseline information for the setting of health priorities and the identification of the need for intervention.

- Intervention programmes for the control of acute pesticide poisoning (including suicide attempts) should be established, monitored, and evaluated.

International agencies should provide support and guidance for the above actions.

Ensuring accurate analysis

Accurate analytical procedures for the monitoring of pesticide exposure, incorporating modern methods of quality assurance, are urgently needed. Work is needed to develop simple, cheap methods based on an appropriate technology.

Epidemiological studies

The identification of the health effects of long-term exposure in the general population is difficult but extremely important.

Every effort should be made to perform epidemiological studies to elucidate this problem, including:

● Improvement of the quality of census, morbidity, and mortality data on a national basis, as well as data on pesticide usage on a local, national, and regional basis.

● Establishment of registers (e.g., for cancer, cardiovascular disease, and birth defects) as these would be of value in studying the relationship between pesticide exposure and disease occurrence.

● Development of geographical mapping methods and other epidemiological techniques to study the relationship between disease and the pattern of pesticide usage on a local, national, and regional basis.

● Identification of occupational groups exposed to pesticides for long periods. Though occupational groups are often exposed to many pesticides in their working life, certain groups of workers may have been exposed to a single pesticide or a single class of pesticides, e.g., organochlorine or organophosphorus compounds; these groups would be of particular importance for studies aimed at refuting or confirming effects shown in animal studies. In addition, specific studies of the effects of defined combined exposures are needed.

REFERENCES

ABOU-DONIA, M. B. & PREISSIG, S. H. (1976a) Delayed neurotoxicity of leptophos: toxic effects on the nervous system of hens. *Toxicology and applied pharmacology*, **35**: 269–282.

ABOU-DONIA, M. B. & PREISSIG, S. H. (1976b) Delayed neurotoxicity from continuous low-dose oral administration of leptophos to hens. *Toxicology and applied pharmacology*, **38**: 595–608.

ADAMS, R. M. (1983) *Occupational skin diseases*. New York, Grune & Stratton.

ALMEIDA, W. F. ET AL. (1978) Influence of nutritional status on the toxicity of food additives and pesticides. In: Galli, C. L. et al., ed., *Chemical toxicology of food*, Amsterdam, Elsevier/North Holland Biomedical Press, pp. 169–184.

ANON (1985) A look at world pesticide markets. *Farm chemicals* (September): 26–34.

BAETJER, A. M. (1983) Water deprivation and food restriction on toxicity of parathion and paraoxon. *Archives of environmental health*, **38**: 168–171.

BAINOVA, A. (1982) Dermal absorption of pesticides. In: *Toxicology of pesticides*, Copenhagen, WHO Regional Office for Europe, pp. 41–53 (European Cooperation on Environmental Health Aspects of the Control of Chemicals, Interim document 9).

BAKER, E. L. JR ET AL. (1978) Epidemic malathion poisoning in Pakistani malaria workers. *Lancet*, **1**: 31–34.

BALK F. & KOEMAN, J. H. (1984) *Future hazards from pesticide use*. Gland, Switzerland, International Union for Conservation of Nature and Natural Resources (Commission on Ecology Papers, No. 6).

BALOCH, U. K. (1985) Problems associated with the use of chemicals by agricultural workers. *Basic life sciences*, **34**: 63–78.

BATES, J. A. R. (1982) Safe practice in pesticide use: pesticide residues in food and the environment. In: *Toxicology of pesticides,* Copenhagen, WHO Regional Office for Europe, pp. 195–213 (European Cooperation on Environmental Health Aspects of the Control of Chemicals, Interim document 9).

BERGER, L. R. (1988) Suicides and pesticides in Sri Lanka. *American journal of public health*, **78**: 826–828.

BOYD, E. M. ET AL. (1969) The effects of diets containing from 0 to 81 percent of casein on the acute oral toxicity of diazinon. *Clinical toxicology*, **2**: 295–301.

BOYD, E. M. ET AL. (1970) Endosulfan toxicity and dietary protein. *Archives of environmental health*, **21**: 15–19.

BULL, D. (1982) *A growing problem: pesticides and the third world poor.* Oxford, OXFAM, 192 pp.

CDFA (1986) *Summary of reports from physicians of illnesses that were reported in California as potentially related to pesticides,* Sacramento, California, California Department of Food and Agriculture.

CHAVEZ, C. T. ET AL. (1985) Methyl bromide optic atrophy. *American journal of ophthalmology*, **99**: 715–719.

CODEX (1984) *Guide to Codex recommendations concerning pesticide residues. Part 1. General notes and guidelines.* The Hague, Codex Alimentarius Commission (Report CAC/PRI-1984).

COPPLESTONE, J. F. (1977) A global view of pesticide safety. In: Watson, D. L. & Brown, A. W. A., ed. *Pesticide management and insecticide resistance,* New York, Academic Press, pp. 147–155.

COPPLESTONE, J. F. (1982) Problems in education on the safe handling of pesticides. In: van Heemstra-Lequin, E. A. H. & Tordoir, W. F., ed. *Education and safe handling in pesticide application,* Amsterdam, Elsevier, pp. 59–64 (Studies in Environmental Science, 18).

COPPLESTONE, J. F. (1985) Pesticide exposure and health in developing countries. In: Turnbull, G. J., ed. *Occupational hazards of pesticide use.* London, Taylor and Francis.

COPPLESTONE, J. F. ET AL. (1976) Exposure to pesticides in agriculture: a survey of spraymen using dimethoate in the Sudan. *Bulletin of the World Health Organization*, **54**: 217–223.

COUNCIL OF EUROPE (1984) *Pesticides—advice and recommendations to be used by national and other authorities as well as manufacturers concerned with the registration of agricultural and non-agricultural pesticides,* 6th ed. Strasbourg, 120 pp.

CSA (1988) Cancer risk of pesticides in agricultural workers. Report by the Council on Scientific Affairs. *Journal of the American Medical Association*, **260**: 959–966.

DAVIES, J. E. (1984) Epidemiologic concerns for exposure assessment. In: Siewierski, M., ed. *Determination and assessment of pesticide exposure,* New York, Elsevier, pp. 67–77 (Studies in Environmental Science, 24).

DAVIES, J. E. ET AL. (1980) Minimizing occupational exposure to pesticides: epidemiological overview. *Residue reviews*, **75**: 7–20.

DAVIES, J. E. ET AL., ed. (1982) *An agrochemical approach to pesticide management: some health and environmental considerations,* Miami, University of Miami, School of Medicine, 320 pp.

DOSSING, M. (1984) Non-invasive assessment of microsomal enzyme activity in occupational medicine: present state of knowledge and future prospectives. *International archives of occupational and environmental health*, **53**: 205–218.

DULOUT, F. N. ET AL. (1985) Sister-chromatide exchanges and chromosomal aberrations in a population exposed to pesticides. *Mutation research*, **143**: 237–244.

EDWARDS, C. A. (1977a) *Impact monitoring of residues from the use of agricultural pesticides in developing countries.* Unpublished document available on request from: Rothamsted Experimental Station, Harpenden, Herts, England.

EDWARDS, C. A. (1977b) Environmental aspects of the usage of pesticides in developing countries. *Mededelingen van de Faculteit Landbouwweten schapper Rijksuniversitet Gent,* **42**(2): 853–868.

EDWARDS, C. A. (1983a) *Environmental pollution by pesticides.* London and New York, Plenum Publishing Company.

EDWARDS, C. A. (1986) Agrochemicals as environmental pollutants. In: van Hofsten, B. & Ekström, G., ed. *Control of pesticide applications and residues in food. A guide and directory 1986,* Uppsala, Swedish Science Press, pp. 1–19.

EDWARDS, C. A. ET AL. (1980) *Pesticide residues in the environment in India.* Bangalore, Raja Press.

ESCAP (1983) *Development/environment trends in Asia and the Pacific: a regional overview.* Bangkok, Committee on Industry, Technology and Human Settlements, Economic and Social Commission of Asia and the Pacific.

ESKENAZI, B. & MAIZLISH, N. A. (1988) Effects of occupational exposure to chemicals on neurobehavioral functioning. In: Tarter R. E. et al., ed. *Neuropsychological disorder in mental illness.* New York, Plenum Press, pp. 223–264.

FAO (1967) *Report of the FAO Panel of Experts on Integrated Pest Control, September 1967.* Rome, Food and Agriculture Organization of the United Nations.

FAO (1977) *Ad hoc government consultation on international standardization of pesticide registration requirements,* Rome, 24–28 October 1977, p. 57 (AGP: 1977/M/9, Appendix IV).

FAO (1979) *Guidelines for integrated control of rice insect pests.* Rome, Food and Agriculture Organization of the United Nations, 115 pp (FAO Plant Production and Protection Paper, No. 14).

FAO (1985a) *Prevention of post-harvest food losses.* Rome, Food and Agriculture Organization of the United Nations, 120 pp.

FAO (1985b) *Guidelines on good labelling practice for pesticides.* Rome, Food and Agriculture Organization of the United Nations.

FAO (1986a) *International code of conduct on the distribution and use of pesticides.* Rome, Food and Agriculture Organization of the United Nations, 28 pp.

FAO (1986b) *FAO production yearbook.* Vol. 39, Rome, Food and Agriculture Organization of the United Nations.

FAO/WHO (1976) *Pesticide residues in food:* report of the 1975 Joint Meeting of the FAO Working Party of Experts on Pesticide Residues and the WHO Expert Committee on Pesticide Residues (WHO Technical Report Series, No. 592; FAO Plant Production and Protection Series, No. 1).

FINKELMAN, J. & MOLINA, G. (1988) [*Pesticides and health. Situation in Latin America.*] Metepec, Mexico, 28 pp. (1988 revision of 1987 report from the Pan American Center for Human Ecology and Health) (in Spanish).

FRIEDMAN, J. M. (1984) Does Agent Orange cause birth defects? *Teratology,* **29**: 193–221.

GEMS (1983) *GEMS/Water data summary.* Burlington, Ontario, Canada Center for Inland Waters.

GEMS (1986) *Chemical contaminants in foods: 1980–1983. Global Environmental Monitoring System.* Unpublished WHO document WHO/EHE/FOS/86.5. Available on request from: Division of Environmental Health, World Health Organization, 1211 Geneva 27, Switzerland.

GIFAP (1988) *Pictograms for agrochemical labels: an aid to the safe handling of pesticides.* Brussels, International Group of National Associations of Manufacturers of Agrochemical Products.

GLOTFELTY, D. E. ET AL. (1987) Pesticides in fog. *Nature (London),* **325**: 602–605.

GREEN, M. B. ET AL. (1977) *Chemicals for crop protection and pest control.* Oxford, Pergamon Press.

GREEN, M. A. ET AL. (1987) An outbreak of watermelon-borne pesticide toxicity. *American journal of public health,* **77**: 1431–1434.

GRIFFITH, J. ET AL. (1985) Pesticide poisonings reported by Florida citrus fieldworkers. *Journal of environmental science and health,* **B20**(6): 701–727.

GUNN, D. L. & STEVENS, J. G. R. (1976) *Pesticides and human welfare.* Oxford, Oxford University Press.

GUPTA, S. K. ET AL. (1984) Health hazards in pesticide formulators exposed to a combination of pesticides. *Indian journal of medical research,* **79**: 666–672.

GUZELIAN, P. S. ET AL. (1980) Liver structure and function in patients poisoned with chlordecone. *Gastroenterology,* **78**: 206–213.

HASSALL, K. A. (1982) *The chemistry of pesticides: their metabolism, mode of action and uses in crop protection.* Weinheim, Verlag Chemie.

HAYES, W. J. Jr (1975) *Toxicology of pesticides.* Baltimore, USA, Williams and Wilkins Co.

HAYES, W. J. Jr (1982) *Pesticides studied in man.* Baltimore, USA, Williams and Wilkins Co.

HAYES, W. J. ET AL. (1978) Organophosphate poisoning in Rhodesia, *South African medical journal,* **54**: 230–234.

HOWARD, J. K. ET AL. (1981) A study of the health of Malaysian plantation workers with particular reference to paraquat spraymen. *British journal of industrial medicine,* **38**: 110–116.

HUNTER, J. ET AL. (1971) Urinary D-glutaric-acid excretion as a test for hepatic enzyme induction in man. *Lancet,* **1**: 572–575.

IARC (1974) *Some organochlorine pesticides.* Lyon, International Agency for Research on Cancer (IARC Monographs on the Evaluation of Carcinogenic Risks to Humans, No. 5).

IARC (1976) *Some carbamates, thiocarbamates and carbazides.* Lyon,

International Agency for Research on Cancer (IARC Monographs on the Evaluation of Carcinogenic Risks to Humans, No. 12).

IARC (1977) *Some fumigants, the herbicides 2,4-D and 2,4,5-T, chlorinated dibenzodioxins and miscellaneous industrial chemicals.* Lyon, International Agency for Research on Cancer (IARC Monographs on the Evaluation of Carcinogenic Risks to Humans, No. 15).

IARC (1979) *Some halogenated hydrocarbons.* Lyon, International Agency for Research on Cancer (IARC Monographs on the Evaluation of Carcinogenic Risks to Humans, No. 20).

IARC (1980) *Long-term and short-term screening assays for carcinogens: a critical appraisal.* Lyon, International Agency for Research on Cancer (IARC Monographs on the Evaluation of Carcinogenic Risks to Humans, Suppl. 2).

IARC (1982) *Chemicals, industrial processes and industries associated with cancer in humans.* Lyon, International Agency for Research on Cancer (IARC Monographs on the Evaluation of Carcinogenic Risks to Humans, Suppl. 4).

IARC (1983) *Miscellaneous pesticides.* Lyon, International Agency for Research on Cancer (IARC Monographs on the Evaluation of Carcinogenic Risks to Humans, No. 30).

IARC (1985) *Allyl compounds, aldehydes, epoxides and peroxides.* Lyon, International Agency for Research on Cancer (IARC Monographs on the Evaluation of Carcinogenic Risks to Humans, No. 36).

IARC (1987) *Some halogenated hydrocarbons and pesticide exposures.* Lyon, International Agency for Research on Cancer (IARC Monographs on the Evaluation of the Carcinogenic Risk of Chemicals to Humans, No. 41).

IARC (1988) *Overall evaluations of carcinogenicity: an updating of IARC monographs, volumes 1–42.* Lyon, International Agency for Research on Cancer (IARC Monographs on the Evaluation of Carcinogenic Risks to Humans, Suppl. 7).

ILO (1977) *Safe use of pesticides.* Geneva, International Labour Office, 42 pp (Occupational Safety and Health Series, Report No. 38).

JEYARATNAM, J. ET AL. (1982) Survey of pesticide poisoning in Sri Lanka. *Bulletin of the World Health Organization,* **60**: 615–619.

JEYARATNAM, J. (1985) 1984 and occupational health in developing countries, *Scandinavian journal of work, environment and health,* **11**: 229–234.

JEYARATNAM, J. ET AL. (1986) Blood cholinesterase levels among agricultural workers in four Asian countries. *Toxicology letters,* **33**: 195–201.

JEYARATNAM, J. ET AL. (1987) Survey of acute pesticide poisoning among agricultural workers in four Asian countries. *Bulletin of the World Health Organization,* **65**: 521–527.

KAGAN, Y. S. (1985) *Principles of pesticide toxicology.* Moscow, USSR Commission for UNEP, Centre of International Projects (GNKT).

KAHN, E. (1976) Pesticide-related illness in California farm workers. *Journal of occupational medicine,* **18**: 693–696.

KALOYANOVA, F. (1982) Evaluation of pesticide toxicity for sanitary registration. In: *Toxicology of pesticides*. Copenhagen, WHO Regional Office for Europe, pp. 265–274 (European Cooperation on Environmental Health Aspects of the Control of Chemicals, Interim document 9).

KALOYANOVA, F. (1983) Interactions of pesticides. In: *Health effects of combined exposures to chemicals in work and community environments*. Copenhagen, WHO Regional Office for Europe, pp. 165–195 (Interim document 11).

KALOYANOVA, F. (1986) [Classification of pesticides by health and environmental hazard.] *Higiena i zdraveopazvane*, **29**: 21–26 (in Bulgarian, with English summary).

KAPOOR, S. K. ET AL. (1980) Contamination of bovine milk with DDT and HCH residues in relation to their usage in malaria control programme. *Journal of environmental science and health*, **B15**(5): 545–557.

KASHYAP, S. K. (1979) *Health implication of pesticides in public health programmes. Proceedings of Indo-US workshop on biodegradable pesticides, 16–17 April 1979, Lucknow*. Available on request from Industrial Toxicology Research Center, Lucknow, India.

KEARNEY, P. C. (1980) Nitrosamines and pesticides. A special report on the occurrence of nitrosamines as terminal residue resulting from agricultural use of certain pesticides. *Pure and applied chemistry*, **53**: 499–526.

KNAPP, L. W. (1982) Safety of pesticide applicators. In: *Toxicology of pesticides*. Copenhagen, WHO Regional Office for Europe, pp. 253–264 (European Cooperation on Environmental Health Aspects of the Control of Chemicals, Interim document 9).

KOLMODIN, B. ET AL. (1969) Effect of environmental factors on drug metabolism: Decreased plasma halflife of antipyrine in workers exposed to chlorinated hydrocarbon insecticides. *Clinical pharmacology and therapeutics*, **10**: 638–642.

KOZLYUK, A. S. ET AL. (1987) [Immunity in children living in regions with different pesticide applications.] *Gigiena i sanitaria*, **6**: 26–28 (in Russian).

KRIJNEN, C. J. & BOYD, E. M. (1970) Susceptibility to captan pesticide of albino rats fed from weaning on diets containing various levels of protein. *Food and cosmetic toxicology*, **8**: 35–42.

KURINNI, A. I. & PILINSKAYA, M. A. (1976) [*Study of pesticides as environmental mutagens.*] Kiev, Naukova Dumka Publ. Co. (in Russian).

LAST, J. M. (1988) *A dictionary of epidemiology*. 2nd ed. Oxford, International Epidemiological Association, Oxford University Press, 141 pp.

LAUG, E. P. ET AL. (1951) Occurrence of DDT in human fat and milk. *Archives of industrial hygiene*, **3**: 245.

LEVINE, R. S. (1986) *Assessment of mortality and morbidity due to unintentional pesticide poisonings*. Unpublished WHO document,

WHO/VBC/86.929. Available on request from: Division of Environmental Health, World Health Organization, 1211 Geneva 27, Switzerland.

LOEVINSOHN, M. E. (1987) Insecticide use and increased mortality in rural central Luzon, Philippines. *Lancet*, 1: 1359–1362.

MACKINTOSH, M. E. ET AL. (1978) A survey of the risk factors associated with organophosphate and carbamate pesticide poisoning. *The Central African journal of medicine*, 24: 41–44.

MAIZLISH, N. ET AL. (1987) A behavioural evaluation of pest control workers with short term, low level exposure to the organophosphate diazinon. *American journal of industrial medicine*, 12: 153–172.

MISRA, U. K. ET AL. (1985) Some observations on the macula of pesticide workers. *Human toxicology,* 4: 135–145.

MORGAN, D. P. (1980) Minimizing occupational exposure to pesticides: acute and chronic effects of pesticides on human health. *Residue reviews*, 75: 97–102.

MOWBRAY, D. L. (1986) Pesticide poisoning in Papua New Guinea and the South Pacific. *Papua New Guinea medical journal,* 29: 131–141.

MOWBRAY, D. L. (1988) *Pesticide use in the South Pacific.* Nairobi, UNEP (UNEP Regional Seas Reports and Studies, No. 89).

MURAKAMI, M. (1987) *Review of organochlorine compounds in human tissues and fluids and associated health effects.* Tsukuba, Japan, National Institute of Environmental Studies, 103 pp (Report B-31-87).

NAS (1987) *Regulating pesticides in food: the Delaney paradox.* Washington, National Academy of Sciences, National Academy Press.

NORDBERG, G. F. & ANDERSEN, O. (1981) Metal interactions in carcinogenesis: enhancement, inhibition. *Environmental health perspectives,* 40: 65–81.

NORÉN, K. (1987) *Studies of organochlorine contaminants in human milk.* Stockholm, Karolinska Institute (Dissertation).

PIMENTEL, D. ET AL. (1980) Environmental and social costs of pesticides: a preliminary assessment. *Oikos,* 34: 126–140.

PLESTINA, R. (1984) *Prevention, diagnosis and treatment of pesticide poisoning.* Unpublished WHO document WHO/VBC/84.889. Available on request from: Division of Environmental Health, World Health Organization, 1211 Geneva 27, Switzerland.

POLCHENKO, V. I. (1974) *The problem of selection of less dangerous pesticides. Proceedings of the Third International Congress of Pesticides Chemistry, Helsinki, 3–9 July 1974,* p. 528. Available on request from International Union of Pure and Applied Chemistry, Templar Square, Cowley, Oxford OX4 3YF, England.

POLCHENKO, V. I. ET AL. (1975) [Comparative incidence of diseases in two rural zones with different intensity of pesticide use.] *Vrachebnoje delo,* 2: 106–108 (in Russian).

RABELLO, M. N. ET AL. (1975) Cytogenetic study on individuals occupationally exposed to DDT. *Mutation research,* 28: 449–454.

REPETTO, R. (1985) *Paying the price: pesticide subsidies in developing countries.* Washington, World Resources Institute, 33 pp (Research Report No. 2).

ROBSON, A. L. ET AL. (1969) Pentachlorophenol poisoning in a nursery for newborn infants. I. Clinical features and treatment. *Journal of pediatrics,* **75**: 309–316.

SAVAGE, E. P. ET AL. (1988) Chronic neurological sequelae of acute organophosphate pesticide poisoning. *Archives of environmental health,* **43**: 38–45.

SENEWIRATNE, B. & THAMBIPILLAI, S. (1974) Pattern of poisoning in a developing agricultural country. *British journal of preventive and social medicine,* **28**: 32–36.

SHARP, D. S. ET AL. (1986) Delayed health hazards of pesticide exposure. *Annual review of public health,* **7**: 441–471.

SHIH, J. H. ET AL. (1985) Prevention of acute parathion and demeton poisoning in farmers around Shanghai, *Scandinavian journal of work, environment and health,* **11** (Suppl. 4): 49–54.

SILANO, V. (1985) *Evaluation of public health hazards associated with chemical accidents.* Toluca, Mexico City, Pan American Center for Human Ecology and Health (ECO).

SINGH, P. D. A. & WEST, M. E. (1985) Acute pesticide poisoning in the Caribbean. *West Indian medical journal,* **34**: 75–83.

SMITH, A. & GRAZ, N. G. (1984) *Urban vector and rodent control services.* Unpublished WHO document WHO/VBC/84.4. Available on request from: Division of Control of Tropical Diseases, World Health Organization, 1211 Geneva 27, Switzerland.

SMITH, A. & LOSSEV, O. (1981) *Pesticides and equipment requirements for national vector control programmes in developing countries 1978–1984.* Unpublished WHO document VBC/81.4. Available on request from: Division of Control of Tropical Diseases, World Health Organization, 1211 Geneva 27, Switzerland.

STARING, W. D. E. (1984) *Pesticides: data collection systems on supply, distribution and use.* Bangkok, United Nations Economic and Social Commission for Asia and the Pacific.

STEENLAND, K. ET AL. (1985) Cytogenic studies in humans after short-term exposure to ethylene dibromide. *Journal of occupational medicine,* **27**: 729–732.

SWEZEY, S. ET AL. (1986) Nicaragua's revolution in pesticide policy. *Environment,* **28**: 6–9 and 29–36.

TAYLOR, J. R. ET AL. (1976) Neurologic disorder induced by kepone: Preliminary report. *Neurology,* **26**: 358–363.

TAYLOR, R. ET AL. (1985) *Paraquat poisoning in Pacific Island countries, 1975–1985.* Noumea, New Caledonia, South Pacific Commission, 58 pp (Technical Paper No. 189).

UNEP (1981) *Agro-industry and the environment. Post harvest loss reduction. Industry and environment,* **4**(1): 1–22.

UNEP/WHO (1987) *Global pollution and health.* Unpublished document.

Available on request from Division of Environmental Health, World Health Organization, 1211 Geneva 27, Switzerland.

UNEP/WHO (1988) *GEMS assessment of freshwater quality.* Unpublished document. Available on request from Division of Environmental Health, World Health Organization, 1211 Geneva 27, Switzerland.

UNIDO (1984) *Report from an Expert Group meeting on quality control of pesticides, Dhaka, Bangladesh 13–17 May 1984.* Regional Network for the Production, Marketing and Control of Pesticides in Asia and the Far East (DP/RAS/82/006, UNIDO/10.594).

WACHTER, A. J. M. & STARING, W. D. E. (1981) *Comparative study on the supply, distribution and use of agropesticides in the ESCAP region.* Bangkok, Agricultural Division, Economic and Social Commission for Asia and the Pacific (Agricultural requisites scheme for Asia and the Pacific, ARSAP/2/Agropesticides).

WARE, G. W. (1983) *Pesticides. Theory and application,* San Francisco, W.H. Freeman and Co..

WEINBACH, E. C. (1957) Biochemical basis for the toxicity of pentachlorophenol. *Proceedings of the national academy of science (USA),* **43**: 393–397.

WHARTON, D. ET AL. (1977) Infertility in male pesticide workers. *Lancet,* **2**: 1259–1261.

WHARTON, D. ET AL. (1979) Testicular function in DBCP exposed pesticide workers. *Journal of occupational medicine,* **21**: 161–166.

WHO (1973) *Safe use of pesticides*: twentieth report of the WHO Expert Committee on Insecticides. Geneva, World Health Organization (WHO Technical Report Series, No. 513).

WHO (1976). Conference on intoxication due to alkylmercury-treated seed, Baghdad, Iraq, 9–13 September 1974. *Bulletin of the World Health Organization,* **53** (Suppl.)

WHO (1978b) *Multilevel course on the safe use of pesticides and on the diagnosis and treatment of pesticide poisoning. Course manual.* Unpublished WHO document WHO/VBC/78.7. Available on request from: Division of Control of Tropical Diseases, World Health Organization, 1211 Geneva 27, Switzerland.

WHO (1979) *DDT and its derivatives.* Geneva, World Health Organization (Environmental Health Criteria, No. 9).

WHO (1980) *National multilevel courses on the safe use of pesticides. Establishment manual.* Unpublished WHO document WHO/VBC/80.1. Available on request from: Division of Control of Tropical Diseases, World Health Organization, 1211 Geneva 27, Switzerland.

WHO (1982a) *Recommended health-based limits in occupational exposure to pesticides*: report of a WHO study group. Geneva, World Health Organization (WHO Technical Report Series, No. 677).

WHO (1982b) *Biological control of vectors of disease*: sixth report of the WHO Expert Committee on Vector Biology and Control. Geneva, World Health Organization (WHO Technical Report Series, No. 679).

WHO (1983) *Integrated vector control*: seventh report of the WHO Expert Committee on Vector Biology and Control. Geneva, World Health Organization (WHO Technical Report Series, No. 688).

WHO (1984a) *2,4-Dichlorophenoxyacetic acid (2,4-D)*. Geneva, World Health Organization (Environmental Health Criteria, No. 29).

WHO (1984b) *Heptachlor*. Geneva, World Health Organization (Environmental Health Criteria, No. 38).

WHO (1984c) *Paraquat and diquat*. Geneva, World Health Organization. (Environmental Health Criteria, No. 39).

WHO (1984d) *Camphechlor*. Geneva, World Health Organization (Environmental Health Criteria, No. 45).

WHO (1984e) *Chemical methods for the control of arthropod vectors and pests of public health importance*. Geneva, World Health Organization, 108 pp.

WHO (1984f) *Guidelines for drinking-water quality. Vol. 1. Recommendations*. Geneva, World Health Organization.

WHO (1985) *Safe use of pesticides*: ninth report of the WHO Expert Committee on Vector Biology and Control. Geneva, World Health Organization (WHO Technical Report Series, No. 720).

WHO (1986a) *Informal consultation on planning strategy for the prevention of pesticide poisoning. Geneva, 25–29 November 1985*. Unpublished WHO document WHO/VBC/86.926. Available on request from: Division of Environmental Health, World Health Organization, 1211 Geneva 27, Switzerland.

WHO (1986b) *Resistance of vectors and reservoirs of disease to pesticides*: tenth report of the WHO Expert Committee on Vector Biology and Control. Geneva, World Health Organization (WHO Technical Report Series, No. 737).

WHO (1986c) *Organophosphorus insecticides: a general introduction*. Geneva, World Health Organization (Environmental Health Criteria, No. 63).

WHO (1986d) *Carbamate pesticides: a general introduction*. Geneva, World Health Organization (Environmental Health Criteria, No. 64).

WHO (1986e) *World health statistics annual*. Geneva, World Health Organization.

WHO (1987a) *Bibliography on health effects of environmental hazards in developing countries*. Unpublished WHO document PEP/87.6. Available on request from: Division of Environmental Health, World Health Organization, 1211 Geneva 27, Switzerland.

WHO (1987b) *Expert group on health hazards in infants associated with exposure to PCBs, dioxins and related compounds in human milk*. Copenhagen, WHO Regional Office for Europe.

WHO (1988a) *Urban vector and pest control*: eleventh report of the WHO Expert Committee on Vector Biology and Control. Geneva, World Health Organization (WHO Technical Report Series, No. 767).

WHO (1988b) *Dithiocarbamate pesticides, ethylenethiourea (ETU), and propylenethiourea (PTU): a general introduction*. Geneva, World Health Organization (Environmental Health Criteria, No. 78).

WHO (1989) *Aldrin and dieldrin*. Geneva, World Health Organization (Environmental Health Criteria, No. 91).

WHO (1990) *The WHO recommended classification of pesticides by hazard, and guidelines to classification 1990–1991*. Unpublished WHO document WHO/PCS/90.1. Available on request from: Division of Environmental Health, World Health Organization, 1211 Geneva 27, Switzerland.

WHO/FAO (1988) *Food irradiation. A technique for preserving and improving the safety of food*. Geneva, World Health Organization.

WOHLFART, D. J. (1981) Paraquat poisoning in Papua New Guinea. *Papua New Guinea medical journal*, **24**(3): 164–168.

WOOD MCKENZIE (1987) *Agrochemical Monitor, No. 50*. London, Wood McKenzie & Co. Ltd., 19 pp.

WORLD BANK (1985) *Guidelines for the selection and use of pesticides in Bank financed projects and their procurement when financed by the Bank*. Washington, DC, World Bank.

WYSOCKI, J. ET AL. (1985) Serum levels of immunoglobulins and C3 component of complement in persons occupationally exposed to chlorinated pesticides. *Medical practitioner*, **36**: 111–117.

XINTARAS, C. ET AL. (1978) *Occupational exposure to leptophos and other chemicals*. Washington, DC, Department of Health, Education and Welfare (Publication No. 78-136).

YODER, J. ET AL. (1973) Lymphocyte chromosome analysis of agricultural workers during extensive occupational exposure to pesticides. *Mutation research*, **21**: 335–340.

ZIELHUIS, R. L. (1972) Epidemiological toxicology of pesticide exposures: report of an international workshop. *Archives of environmental health*, **25**: 399–405.

Annex 1

Global production and use of pesticides

Table A1.1. Annual production of selected pesticides

Pesticide	Annual production, production area, year ((?) = uncertain figure)	Number of suppliers 1986[a]	Source[b]
aldicarb	figures not available	2	
aldrin	4000–5000 tonnes, USA, 1962 4500 tonnes, USA, 1971	5	IARC (1974)
aldrin and dieldrin	20 000 tonnes, total world, 1971 13 000 tonnes, total world, 1972 2500 tonnes, total world, 1984	6	WHO (1989)
dieldrin	2300–4500 tonnes, USA, 1964 450 tonnes, USA, 1971	3	IARC (1974)
endrin	2300–4500 tonnes, USA, 1962 <450 tonnes, USA, 1971	1	IARC (1974)
campheclor (toxaphene)	19 000 tonnes, USA, 1976 27 000 tonnes, USA, 1975	3	IARC (1979)
	34 200 tonnes, USA, 1974 (?)		WHO (1984b)
chlordane	9500 tonnes, USA, 1974	7	IARC (1979)
DDT	82 000 tonnes, USA, 1963 56 000 tonnes, USA, 1969 20 000 tonnes, USA, 1971 39 000 tonnes, USA, 1972 3000 tonnes, Brazil, 1969 350 tonnes, Israel, 1970 4000 tonnes, India, 1971–72 4600 tonnes, Japan, 1970	3	IARC (1974)
	4366 tonnes, USA, 1944 15 079 tonnes, USA, 1945 81 154 tonnes, USA, 1963 60 000 tonnes, total world, 1974		WHO (1979)
ethylene dibromide	150 000 tonnes, USA, 1974 3000–30 000 tonnes, total Benelux, France, Italy, Spain, Switzerland, UK 1974(?) 40 000 tonnes, Europe, 1974 1400 tonnes, Japan, 1975	0	IARC (1977)

Table A1.1   (continued)

Pesticide	Annual production, production area, year ((?) = uncertain figure)	Number of suppliers 1986[a]	Source[b]
HCH (BHC)	53 000 tonnes, USA, 1951 3000 tonnes, USA, 1963 35 400 tonnes, Japan, 1969 2000 tonnes, Japan, 1970 6800 tonnes, Brazil, 1969 2700 tonnes, Brazil, 1965 11 500 tonnes, India, 1968 54 000–64 000 tonnes, world total, 1968	1	IARC (1974)
	30 000 tonnes, France (?) 16 000 tonnes, Federal Republic of Germany (?) 8500 tonnes, Spain (?) 18 000 tonnes, USSR (?)		IARC (1979)
heptachlor	<2300 tonnes, USA, 1962 2700 tonnes, USA, 1971	2	IARC (1974)
	4500 tonnes, USA, July 1975–December 1976		IARC (1979)
lindane	8000 tonnes, USA, 1951 800 tonnes, USA, 1963 4500–5400 tonnes, world total, 1968 500 tonnes, USA, 1964 1300 tonnes, Japan, 1970	30	IARC (1974)
	227 tonnes, USA, 1972 3500 tonnes, France (?) 1700 tonnes, Federal Republic of Germany (?) 1000 tonnes, Spain (?) 2000 tonnes, USSR (?)		IARC (1979)
mirex	454 tonnes, USA, 1971	0	IARC (1974)
	400 tonnes, USA, 1959–1975		WHO (1984a)
paraquat	figures not available	7	
parathion	6400 tonnes, USA, 1972 29 000 tonnes (parathion + methyl parathion), USA, 1983 2000–5000 tonnes, Western Europe (?) 1.2 tonnes, India, 1980–81	7	IARC (1983)
pentachloro-phenol	20 000–23 000 tonnes, USA, annually 1967–1976 14 500 tonnes, Japan, 1966 3300 tonnes, Japan, 1971	4	IARC (1979)
	21 400 tonnes, USA, 1974 22 200 tonnes, USA, 1979 3000 tonnes, USA, 1978 14 500 tonnes, Japan, 1966		IARC (1986)

Table A1.1 (continued)

Pesticide	Annual production, production area, year ((?) = uncertain figure)	Number of suppliers 1986[a]	Source[b]
2,4,5-T	7900 tonnes, USA, 1968 2300 tonnes, USA, 1969	2	IARC (1977)
	5700 tonnes, USA, 1975		IARC (1986)
	2000–20 000 tonnes, Federal Republic of Germany, Spain, UK (?) 4500 tonnes, Federal Republic of Germany, UK (?)		IARC (1977)

[a] Calculated from *International pesticide directory*, 6th ed. (Supplement to *International pest control,* September/October 1986).
[b] Information from publications of the International Agency for Research on Cancer (IARC), Lyon, or the World Health Organization, Geneva, as follows:
  IARC (1974) *Some organochlorine pesticides* (IARC Monographs on the Evaluation of Carcinogenic Risks to Humans, No. 5).
  IARC (1977) *Some fumigants, the herbicides 2, 4-D and 2,4,5-T, chlorinated dibenzodioxins and miscellaneous industrial chemicals* (IARC Monographs on the Evaluation of Carcinogenic Risks to Humans, No. 15).
  IARC (1979) *Some halogenated hydrocarbons* (IARC Monographs on the Evaluation of Carcinogenic Risks to Humans, No. 20).
  IARC (1983) *Miscellaneous pesticides* (IARC Monographs on the Evaluation of Carcinogenic Risks to Humans, No. 30).
  IARC (1986) *Some halogenated hydrocarbons and pesticide exposures* (IARC Monographs on the Evaluation of Carcinogenic Risks to Humans, No. 41).
  WHO (1979) *DDT and its derivatives* (Environmental Health Criteria, No. 9).
  WHO (1984a) *Mirex* (Environmental Health Criteria, No. 44).
  WHO (1984b) *Camphechlor* (Environmental Health Criteria, No. 45).
  WHO (1989) *Aldrin and dieldrin* (Environmental Health Criteria, No. 91).

Table A1.2. The herbicide market by crop, 1985 (million US
dollars, 1984)[a]

Crop	USA	Western Europe	East Asia	Rest of world	Total
Maize	1034	118	18	225	1395
Cotton	125	7	13	143	288
Wheat	148	439	28	176	791
Sorghum	79	8	3	12	102
Rice	60	23	334	90	507
Other grains	40	245	17	115	417
Soya beans	1095	13	21	219	1348
Tobacco	17	3	3	7	30
Peanuts (groundnuts)	33	–	5	8	46
Sugar beet	24	204	5	54	287
Sugar cane	15	–	14	119	148
Coffee	–	–	6	23	29
Cocoa	–	–	1	11	12
Tea	–	–	9	13	22
Rubber	–	–	55	10	65
Other field crops	25	61	50	53	189
Alfalfa	18	12	1	3	34
Other hay and forage	8	8	1	1	18
Pasture and rangeland	51	12	9	44	116
Fruits, vegetables, and horticultural crops	142	193	71	81	487
Total	2914	1346	664	1407	6331
%	46	21	10	22	100

[a] Source: A look at world pesticide markets. *Farm chemicals*, (September): 26–34
(1985). (Reproduced by permission.)

Table A1.3. The insecticide market by crop, 1985 (million US dollars, 1984)[a]

Crop	USA	Western Europe	East Asia	Rest of world	Total
Maize	262	70	28	96	456
Cotton	206	24	149	590	969
Wheat	16	34	23	35	108
Sorghum	20	6	6	24	56
Rice	24	7	498	104	633
Other grains	7	22	5	12	46
Soya beans	30	4	27	67	128
Tobacco	33	8	31	38	108
Peanuts (groundnuts)	22	1	19	23	65
Sugar beet	8	59	6	24	97
Sugar cane	6	–	9	27	42
Coffee	–	–	5	39	44
Cocoa	–	–	13	25	38
Tea	–	–	38	19	57
Rubber	–	–	11	8	19
Other field crops	22	43	45	60	170
Alfalfa	18	8	2	4	32
Other hay and forage	2	3	2	6	13
Pasture and rangeland	6	2	2	9	19
Fruits, vegetables, and horticultural crops	299	213	329	327	1168
Total	981	504	1248	1535	4268
%	23	12	29	36	100

[a] Source: A look at world pesticide markets. *Farm chemicals*, (September): 26–34 (1985). (Reproduced by permission.)

Table A1.4. The fungicide market by crop, 1985 (million US dollars, 1984)[a]

Crop	USA	Western Europe	East Asia	Rest of world	Total
Maize	36	23	18	40	116
Cotton	11	1	3	8	23
Wheat	12	284	6	49	351
Sorghum	2	3	2	5	12
Rice	7	2	250	47	302
Other grains	5	118	5	21	149
Soya beans	18	1	4	6	28
Tobacco	15	4	10	11	39
Peanuts (groundnuts)	45	–	5	6	55
Sugar beet	7	12	5	25	49
Sugar cane	2	–	3	21	26
Coffee	–	–	5	41	46
Cocoa	–	–	3	10	13
Tea	–	–	13	5	18
Rubber	–	–	9	3	12
Other field crops	4	21	8	8	50
Alfalfa	2	2	–	4	8
Other hay and forage	1	1	1	2	5
Pasture and rangeland	1	–	1	1	3
Fruits, vegetables, and horticultural crops	145	571	218	299	1232
Total	313	1043	569	612	2537
%	12	41	22	24	100

[a] Source: A look at world pesticide markets. *Farm chemicals,* (September): 26–34 (1985). (Reproduced by permission.)

Use and choice of individual pesticides based on recommended restrictions on availability

This annex contains information on the main uses of, and hazard classification for, a number of selected pesticides. Recommended restrictions on availability are given for pesticides covered by FAO/WHO Data Sheets on Pesticides. Asterisks show that restricted availability of a pesticide has been recommended; the more asterisks the more stringent the restrictions that are recommended. By comparing pesticides with the same main use, the least hazardous pesticide can sometimes be selected.

Basis of classification

The classification used by WHO (see Table 16, page 42) distinguishes between the more and the less hazardous forms of each pesticide, in that it is based on the toxicity of the technical compound and its formulation. In particular, allowance is made for the lesser hazards of solid formulations as compared with liquids.

The classification is based primarily on the acute oral and dermal toxicity for the rat, since determination of these values is standard procedure in toxicology. Where the dermal LD_{50} of a compound would place it in a more restrictive class than the oral LD_{50}, the compound is always classified in the more restrictive category. Provision is made for the classification of a particular compound to be adjusted if, for any reason, the acute hazard to man is found to differ from that indicated by LD_{50} assessment alone.

The present WHO classification includes the category "unlikely to present acute hazard in normal use" (class 0) in addition to the four categories in Table 16. This category is used for pesticides recognized as potential causes of health effects (e.g., benomyl), but for which these effects are unlikely to occur. The oral LD_{50} for class 0 pesticides should be over 2000 mg/kg of body weight (solids) or over 3000 mg/kg of body weight (liquids).

Alternative systems of hazard classification that take into account long-term effects include those of the USSR[a] and Bulgaria.[b]

Use categories and recommended restrictions on availability

The use categories set out in Table A2.1 do not prohibit the use of a very highly toxic compound. Such prohibition may be desirable if control measures cannot be enforced to the extent that safety in the use of the compound can be assured. However, this is a matter for national decision in the light of prevailing circumstances.

Table A2.1. Use categories of pesticides according to recommended restrictions on availability[a]

Category 1 ****	Pesticides in this category should be available only to professional operators, individually licensed, who have demonstrated a good knowledge of the chemical, its uses and hazards, and the precautions to be taken in use. This category includes only a few very highly toxic pesticides.
Category 2 ***	Pesticides in this category should be available only to contractors, pest control operators, etc., who will apply the pesticide under strictly controlled and supervised conditions, using trained operators. The application of pesticides will normally be the major part of their commercial operation. This category includes most of the very highly toxic pesticides and other pesticides for which it is felt that special training or supervision in use is necessary.
Category 3 **	Pesticides in this category should be available to commercial applicators (farmers, fruit growers, foresters, fishermen, etc., and those responsible for bulk food storage), for whom the application of a pesticide is not necessarily a major part of their operations, subject to a permit being received from a competent authority, specifying the pesticide, conditions of use, and the precautions to be taken. This category includes pesticides that are highly toxic, and those that have an adverse effect on the environment to the extent that their uncontrolled use without permit is undesirable.
Category 4 *	Pesticides in this category should be available in the same manner as those in category 3, but without the requirement that a permit be issued. This category includes toxic pesticides that may be distributed for commercial use, but should not be available to the general public.
Category 5	Pesticides in this category may be made available to the general public for specified uses. This category applies to all pesticides or their formulations not included in categories 1–4.

[a] Source: WHO/FAO. *Introduction to data sheets.* Unpublished WHO document VBC/DS/75.0. Available on request from: Division of Environmental Health, World Health Organization, 1211 Geneva 27, Switzerland.

[a] Kagan, Y. S. *Principles of pesticide toxicology.* Moscow, USSR Commission for UNEP, Centre of International Projects (GNKT), 1985.
[b] Kaloyanova, F. Evaluation of pesticide toxicity for sanitary registration. In: *Toxicology of pesticides.* Copenhagen, WHO Regional Office for Europe, 1982 (European Cooperation on Environmental Health Aspects of the Control of Chemicals, Interim document 9).

Table A2.2. Use and choice of individual pesticides based on recommended restrictions on availability[a]

Pesticide	Main use[b]	WHO hazard classification of active ingredient	FAO/WHO recommended restrictions on availability of formulations (see Table A2.1)
acephate	I	III	–
aldicarb	I-S	Ia	All formulations (1983): ***
aldrin	I	Ib	Liquid formulations over 25%: ** Liquid formulations over 2.5% and solid formulations over 10%: * All other formulations: category 5
azinphos-methyl	I	Ib	Liquid formulations 8% and above: *** Other liquid formulations: ** Solid formulations 32% and above: *** Other solid formulations: **
bendiocarb	I	II	Solid formulations over 10%: ** Other solid formulations: *
benomyl	F	0	
bioresmethrin	I	0	All formulations (1978): category 5
bis (tributyltin) oxide	F, M	Ib	Liquid formulations over 10%: ** Other liquid formulations: *
brodifacoum	R	Ia	All available (1984) solid formulations (baits) 0.005% or less: category 5
camphechlor	I	II	Liquid formulations over 50%: ** Liquid formulations over 5% and solid formulations over 20%: * All other formulations: category 5
captan	F	0	All formulations: category 5
carbaryl	I	II	Liquids 250 g/l or more: * All other formulations: category 5
carbendazim	F	0	–
carbofuran	I	Ib	Liquid formulations 4% and above: *** Other liquid formulations: ** Solid formulations 16% and above: *** Other solid formulations: **
cartap	I	II	–
chlordane	I	II	All formulations over 10%: ** All formulations 10% or less: category 5
chlordimeform	F	II	–
chlorophacinone	R	Ia	All formulations: * or category 5
chlorphoxim	I	0	Liquid formulations 20% and above and solid formulations over 40%: * All other formulations: category 5
chlorpyrifos	I	II	Liquid formulations over 50%: ** Liquid formulations over 5% and solid formulations over 20%: * All other formulations: category 5
chlorpyrifos methyl	I	0	Liquid formulations 25% and above: * All other formulations: category 5
cypermethrin	I	II	Liquid formulations over 15%: ** Other liquid formulations: *

125

Table A2.2 (continued)

Pesticide	Main use[b]	WHO hazard classification of active ingredient	FAO/WHO recommended restrictions on availability of formulations (see Table A2.1)
2,4-D	H	II	All formulations over 10%: * All formulations 10% or less: category 5
DBCP	F-S	Ia	–
DDT	I	II	Solid formulations 10% and over and all liquid formulations over 2%: * Solid formulations below 10%: category 5
deltamethrin	I	II	All liquid formulations over 20% (1984): * All other formulations: category 5
demeton-S-methyl	I	Ib	Liquid formulations 20% and above: *** Other liquid formulations: **
diazinon	I	II	Liquid formulations over 20%: ** Other liquid formulations and solid formulations over 50%: * All other solid formulations: category 5
dichlorvos	I	Ib	Liquid formulations over 30%: ** Liquid formulations over 3% and solid formulations over 12%, except slow release formulations: * Other formulations: category 5
difenzoquat	H	II	–
dimethoate	I	II	Liquid formulations 10% and above: ** Liquid formulations below 10%: * Solid formulations over 25%: ** All other formulations: *
diquat	H	II	Formulations over 5%: * Formulations 5% or below: category 5
endosulfan	I	II	Liquid formulations over 5%: ** All other liquid formulation and solid formulations over 20%: * All other formulations: category 5
endrin	I	Ib	Liquid and solid formulations over 10%: *** All other formulations: **
fenitrothion	I	II	All formulations 10% or above: * Formulations below 10%: category 5
fensulfothion	I, N	Ia	Liquid formulations above 15%: *** All other liquid formulations and solid formulations 10% or above: ** All other formulations: *
fenthion	I, L	Ib	Liquid formulations over 10%: ** All other liquid formulations and solid formulations over 10%: * All other formulations: category 5
fentin compounds	F	II	Formulations 10% and above: * Formulations below 10%: category 5
glyphosate	H	0	–
guazatine	FST	II	–

126

Table A2.2   (continued)

Pesticide	Main use[b]	WHO hazard classification of active ingredient	FAO/WHO recommended restrictions on availability of formulations (see Table A2.1)
heptachlor	I	II	Liquid formulations 50% or above: ✱✱ Liquid formulations over 5% and solid formulations over 20%: ✱ All other formulations: category 5
hexachlorobenzene	FST	Ia	All formulations: ✱✱
jodfenphos	I	0	Liquid and solid formulations over 10%: ✱ Other formulations: category 5
leptophos	I	Ia	Granular formulations below 2%: category 5 All other formulations: ✱✱✱✱
lindane	I	II	Liquid formulations over 50%: ✱✱ Liquid formulations over 5% and solid formulations over 20%: ✱ All other formulations: category 5
linuron	H	0	–
malathion	I	III	Formulations 2% and above: ✱ Formulations below 2%: category 5
mecoprop	H	III	
methomyl	I	Ib	Liquid formulations 8.5% and above: ✱✱✱ Other liquid formulations: ✱✱ Solid formulations 35% and above: ✱✱✱ Other solid formulations 3.5% and above: ✱✱
methoprene	IGR	0	All formulations: category 5
methoxychlor	I	0	All formulations over 10%: ✱ All formulations 10% or below: category 5
methyl bromide	I(FM)	NC[c]	All formulations: ✱✱
mevinphos	I	Ia	Liquid formulations over 20%: ✱✱✱ Liquid formulations over 2% and solid formulations over 20%: ✱✱ All other formulations: ✱
monocrotophos	I	Ib	–
naled	I	II	All formulations over 5%: ✱✱ All formulations 5% or below: ✱
oxamyl	I	Ib	Liquid formulations 24% (1983): ✱✱✱ Solid (granular) formulations of 10% (1983): ✱✱
paraquat	H	II	Liquid formulations 10% or above and solids over 25%: ✱ All other formulations: category 5
parathion	I	Ia	All formulations: ✱ or ✱✱
parathion-methyl	I	Ia	All formulations: ✱✱
pentachlorophenol	I H	Ib	–
permethrin	I	II	All formulations (1984): category 5

Table A2.2   (continued)

Pesticide	Main use[b]	WHO hazard classification of active ingredient	FAO/WHO recommended restrictions on availability of formulations (see Table A2.1)
phenthoate	I	II	Liquid formulations over 20%: ** Other liquid formulations and solid formulations over 8%: * All other solid formulations: category 5
phosalone	I	II	–
phosphine	I(FM)R	NC[c]	All formulations: ***
phoxim	I	II	80% ULV concentrate: ** Other liquid formulations over 25% and solid formulations over 40%: * All other formulations of lower concentration: category 5
pirimiphos methyl	I	III	Liquid formulations over 10% and solid formulations over 30%: * Other formulations: category 5
propoxur	I	II	Liquid formulations over 50%: ** Liquid formulations over 5% and solid formulations over 20%: * All other formulations: category 5
pyrethrins	I	II	Liquid formulations over 50%: * All other formulations: category 5
sodium fluoroacetate	R	Ia	Solid formulations over 10% and liquid formulations over 1%: **** Solid formulations over 5%: *** Solid formulations over 0.5%: **
2,4,5-T	H	II	Liquid formulations over 25% and neat solid formulations: * All other formulations: category 5
temephos	I	0	All formulations: category 5
thallium sulfate	R, I	Ib	All formulations: ***
trichlorfon	I	III	Formulations 2% and above: * Formulations below 2%: category 5
trifenmorph	M	III	All available formulations (1985): category 5
warfarin	R	Ib	Pre-prepared baits: category 5 All other formulations: *
zinc phosphide	R	Ib	All formulations: ***

[a] Sources: FAO/WHO data sheets on pesticides and *The WHO recommended classification of pesticides by hazard and guidelines to classification, 1990–1991.* Unpublished WHO document WHO/PCS/90.1; available on request from Division of Environmental Health, World Health Organization, 1211 Geneva 27, Switzerland.
[b] In most cases, a single use is given; this is for identification purposes only and does not exclude other uses: F, fungicide; FM, fumigant; FST, fungicide for seed treatment; H, herbicide; I, insecticide; IGR, insect growth regulator; L, larvicide; M, molluscicide; N, nematocide; R, rodenticide; -S, applied to soil (not used with herbicides or plant growth regulators).
[c] Not classified.